Camberwell Assessment of Need for the Elderly

Camberwell Assessment of Need for the Elderly (CANE)

Edited by

Juanita Hoe
City, University of London

Martin Orrell
University of Nottingham

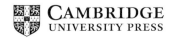
CAMBRIDGE
UNIVERSITY PRESS

CAMBRIDGE
UNIVERSITY PRESS

University Printing House, Cambridge CB2 8BS, United Kingdom

One Liberty Plaza, 20th Floor, New York, NY 10006, USA

477 Williamstown Road, Port Melbourne, VIC 3207, Australia

314–321, 3rd Floor, Plot 3, Splendor Forum, Jasola District Centre, New Delhi – 110025, India

103 Penang Road, #05-06/07, Visioncrest Commercial, Singapore 238467

Cambridge University Press is part of the University of Cambridge.

It furthers the University's mission by disseminating knowledge in the pursuit of
education, learning, and research at the highest international levels of excellence.

www.cambridge.org
Information on this title: www.cambridge.org/9781911623366
DOI: 10.1017/9781911623373

First published 2021

Printed in the United Kingdom by TJ Books Limited, Padstow Cornwall

A catalogue record for this publication is available from the British Library.

ISBN 978-1-911-62336-6 Paperback

Contents

List of Figures   vi
List of Tables   vii
List of Contributors   viii
Acknowledgements   x

1   **An Introduction to Needs Assessment and Use of the Camberwell Assessment of Need for the Elderly**   1
Kunle Ashaye, Dilini Jayalath and Juanita Hoe

2   **Self-Reported Needs of People with Dementia Living at Home: A Scoping Review**   10
Alžběta Bártová, Iva Holmerová, Vladimíra Dostálová, Hana Bláhová and Michal Šteffl

3   **Needs of Older Primary Care Patients**   20
Janine Stein and Steffi Gerlinde Riedel-Heller

4   **Unmet Needs of Older People with and Without Depression in Residential Homes**   34
Hein van Hout, Jannicke M. Iversen and Marijke Boorsma

5   **Needs of Older People Living Alone: A Critical Review**   44
Raffaela Carvacho and Claudia Miranda-Castillo

6   **Needs Assessment of People with Dementia and Impact of Caregiver Burden**   52
Myonghwa Park, Thi-Thanh-Tinh Giap, Miri Jeong, Younghye Go and Dong Young Lee

7   **Crisis and Assessment of Need in Dementia: Development of a Home Treatment Package**   62
Juanita Hoe, Ritchard Ledgerd, Sandeep Toot and Martin Orrell

8   **Needs of People with Young-Onset Dementia**   77
Christian Bakker and Britt Appelhof

9   **Needs of Older People in Long-Term Care Settings**   86
Justyna Mazurek, Dorota Szcześniak and Joanna Rymaszewska

10   **Needs and Healthcare Costs in Old Age: An Application of the Camberwell Assessment of Need for the Elderly**   91
André Hajek, Janine Stein and Hans-Helmut König

11   **The Future of Needs Assessment Research**   97
Juanita Hoe and Martin Orrell

12   **Instructions for the CANE**   105

Index   141

Figures

2.1 Search flowchart in accordance with PRISMA guidelines   11

3.1 Distribution of unmet needs from the patients´ perspective ($n = 231$)   24

3.2 Ten most frequently rated unmet needs from the patients´ perspective across the four disease-specific subgroups   25

3.3 Ten most frequently rated unmet needs from the relatives´ perspective across the four disease-specific subgroups   26

3.4 Ten most frequently rated unmet needs from the GPs´ perspective across the four disease-specific subgroups   27

4.1 Sample derivation   35

4.2 Percentages of unmet needs in CANE categories among depressed and non-depressed persons   40

5.1 Study selection process   46

6.1 Unmet needs with highest rate according to burden groups ($n = 320$)   58

6.2 Number of unmet needs and burden score according to different groups of number of unmet needs ($n = 320$)   58

7.1 Consultation and consensus processes used to develop the home treatment package   66

7.2 Home treatment package advisory protocol pathway   71

9.1 Profile of an older person staying in a long-term care setting   87

Tables

1.1 Items Included in the Camberwell Assessment of Need for the Elderly 2

2.1 Summary of Articles Used in Thematic Analysis 12

3.1 Socio-demographic Characteristics of Patients 23

4.1 Description of the Total Study Population ($n = 213$) and for Persons Who Are Depressed or Non-depressed 36

4.2 Total Needs and Respectively Met and Unmet Needs (CANE) Separately for the Total Group of Persons in Residential Homes ($n = 213$) 37

4.3 Needs Measured by CANE Among Persons Who Are Depressed or Non-depressed 39

4.4 Unmet Needs (CANE) Among Persons Who Are Depressed or Non-depressed 41

5.1 Characteristics of Selected Studies 47

6.1 Characteristics of the People with Dementia and Their Family Caregivers 54

6.2 Needs of People with Dementia and the Source of Help They Received ($n = 320$) 55

6.3 Burden on Family Caregivers of People with Dementia ($n = 320$) 57

7.1 Example of Interventions for the Problem Areas Contributing to Crises in Dementia (Behavioural/Psychological Domain) 67

7.2 Categorisation of the CANE Items to the Five Critical Domains that Contribute to Crises 68

10.1 Sample Characteristics ($n = 1,095$) 93

10.2 Determinants of Total Healthcare Costs (Societal Perspective): Results of Regression Analysis (Generalised Linear Models with Log Link and Gamma Distribution) 94

Contributors

Britt Appelhof

Radboud University Medical Centre, Department of Primary and Community Care, Radboudumc Alzheimer Centre, Nijmegen, Netherlands, and Archipel, Centre for Geriatric Care, Eindhoven, Netherlands

Kunle Ashaye

Mental Health Services for Older People, Hertfordshire Partnership University, National Health Service Foundation Trust, London, United Kingdom

Christian Bakker

Radboud University Medical Centre, Department of Primary and Community Care, Radboudumc Alzheimer Centre, Nijmegen, Netherlands; Groenhuysen, Center for Geriatric Care, Roosendaal, Netherlands; and Dutch Young-Onset Dementia Knowledge Centre, Amersfoort, Netherlands

Alžběta Bártová

Department of Longevity Studies, Faculty of Humanities, Charles University, Prague, Czech Republic

Hana Bláhová

Department of Longevity Studies, Faculty of Humanities, Charles University, Prague, Czech Republic

Marijke Boorsma

Amsterdam University Medical Centres, Vrije University, and Department of General Practice, Amsterdam Public Health Institute, Amsterdam, Netherlands

Raffaela Carvacho

Millennium Institute for Research in Depression and Personality and the Pontificia Universidad Católica de Chile, School of Psychology, Santiago, Chile

Vladimíra Dostálová

Department of Longevity Studies, Faculty of Humanities, Charles University, Prague, Czech Republic

Thi-Thanh-Tinh Giap

Research and Education Centre for Evidence-Based Nursing Knowledge, College of Nursing, Chungnam National University, Daejeon, Republic of Korea

Younghye Go

Research and Education Centre for Evidence-Based Nursing Knowledge, College of Nursing, Chungnam National University, Daejeon, Republic of Korea

André Hajek

Department of Health Economics and Health Services Research, University Medical Center Hamburg-Eppendorf, Hamburg Centre for Health Economics, Hamburg, Germany

Juanita Hoe

Division of Nursing, School of Health Sciences, City, University of London, London, United Kingdom

Iva Holmerová

Department of Longevity Studies, Faculty of Humanities, Charles University, Prague, Czech Republic

Jannicke M. Iversen

Amsterdam University Medical Centres, Vrije University, and Department of General Practice, Amsterdam Public Health Institute, Amsterdam, Netherlands

Dilini Jayalath

Mental Health Services for Older People, Hertfordshire Partnership University, National Health Service Foundation Trust, London, United Kingdom

Miri Jeong

Research and Education Center for Evidence-Based Nursing Knowledge, College of Nursing, Chungnam National University, Daejeon, Republic of Korea

Hans-Helmut König

Department of Health Economics and Health Services Research, University Medical Center Hamburg-Eppendorf, Hamburg Centre for Health Economics, Hamburg, Germany

Dong Young Lee
Department of Neuropsychiatry, Seoul National University Hospital, Seoul, Republic of Korea

Ritchard Ledgerd
Dementia Care Research Centre, North East London National Health Service Foundation Trust, London, United Kingdom

Justyna Mazurek
Department and Division of Medical Rehabilitation, Wroclaw Medical University, Wroclaw, Poland

Claudia Miranda-Castillo
Faculty of Nursing, Universidad Andres Bello and Millennium Institute for Research in Depression and Personality, Santiago, Chile

Martin Orrell
Division of Psychiatry and Applied Psychology, Faculty of Medicine and Health Sciences, Institute of Mental Health, University of Nottingham, Nottingham, United Kingdom

Myonghwa Park
Research and Education Center for Evidence-Based Nursing Knowledge, College of Nursing, Chungnam National University, Daejeon, Republic of Korea

Steffi Gerlinde Riedel-Heller
Medical Faculty, Institute of Social Medicine, Occupational Health and Public Health,

University of Leipzig, Leipzig, Germany

Joanna Rymaszewska
Department of Psychiatry, Wroclaw Medical University, Wroclaw, Poland

Michal Šteffl
Department of Longevity Studies, Faculty of Humanities, Charles University, Prague, Czech Republic

Janine Stein
Medical Faculty, Institute of Social Medicine, Occupational Health and Public Health, University of Leipzig, Leipzig, Germany

Dorota Szcześniak
Division of Psychotherapy and Psychosomatic Medicine, Department of Psychiatry, Wroclaw Medical University, Wroclaw, Poland

Sandeep Toot
Dementia Care Research Centre, North East London National Health Service Foundation Trust, London, United Kingdom

Hein van Hout
Amsterdam University Medical Centres, Vrije University, and Department of General Practice, Amsterdam Public Health Institute, Amsterdam, Netherlands

Acknowledgements

Firstly, we would like to thank Cambridge University Press for the opportunity to write this second edition of the *Camberwell Assessment of Need for the Elderly (CANE)*. The first paper on the CANE was published in 2000, followed by publication of the first edition of the Camberwell Assessment of Need for the Elderly (CANE), in 2004. Preparing this second edition has given us time to examine 20 years' worth of needs assessment research using the CANE with older people, which has been an enlightening and informative task. The growth in studies using the CANE is encouraging and has helped highlight the potential for future research and use of needs assessment as a health outcome measure. Particularly evident is the need to develop and evaluate interventions that can be used to successfully meet the unmet needs of older people identified within these studies.

We would like to thank all the authors who have contributed chapters to this book and have provided us with new research and insightful perspectives on how the CANE has been or can be used to assess the needs of older people in a variety of contexts. We would also like to extend our appreciation to the many academics and clinicians who have published research showing the effectiveness of using the CANE within such a diverse range of older populations across the world. We would especially like to thank all the participants and their families for their involvement in the published studies about needs assessment research in older people. Mostly, thank you to all for helping to build the evidence base around needs assessment, which can be used to find ways to improve services and care for older people.

Finally, for help with preparing this second edition for publication, we send a special thanks to Chrissy Bailey, business support officer at the Institute of Mental Health, University of Nottingham, for her proficient administrative support and to Elena Profyri, a researcher at City, University of London, for her excellent editing and proofing skills. We also thank Monica Manela and Lucy Webster, two researchers at University College London who helped with updating the prompts and reviewing the terminology used in the CANE assessment to ensure that these reflect more present-day language and contemporary issues impacting older people's lives. Your contributions have all been invaluable in preparing this work for publication.

An Introduction to Needs Assessment and Use of the Camberwell Assessment of Need for the Elderly

Kunle Ashaye, Dilini Jayalath and Juanita Hoe

1.1 Introduction

Needs assessment is a systematic approach to identifying the health and healthcare needs of a population that allows services to make changes to improve health service delivery.[1] Detecting unmet needs enables gaps in service provision to be recognised and for health policy to introduce changes that can reduce health inequalities and improve health outcomes.[2] Equally, identifying areas of met needs means that the effectiveness of service delivery can be evaluated. With the rising cost of healthcare, the use of needs assessment has risen in prominence as it can aid decision-making in the planning of resources.[3]

The world's population is ageing, and older age is associated with increased risk of co-morbidity, disability and frailty. As people age, their care needs tend to become more complex with increasing dependency on others, and they are more likely to require care.[4] It is therefore essential that their health needs are assessed and responded to in a more holistic way, which can help older people to live independently and achieve a good quality of life. Care, in essence, is a fulfilment of needs and includes requirements that are unique to each individual. It should be planned well ahead and before reaching a stage where it becomes impractical to meet the needs that are apparent. Currently, UK health and social care services are inadequately designed to meet the needs of older people with multiple and complex chronic health conditions.[5] In addition, publicly funded health and social care has become increasingly restricted to those with complex health or substantial and critical social care needs as services struggle to keep pace with the demands of the ageing population.[6] The United Nations issued a call for governments to design innovative policies and public services specifically targeted to older people that address housing, employment, healthcare, infrastructure and social protection.[7] Consequently, being able to reliably identify the integrated health, social and environmental needs of older people has become paramount. The ability to conduct comprehensive and effective needs assessment ensures that services can be adapted and organised to meet the identified needs of older populations.

1.2 Needs Assessment and Older People

At an individual level, assessment of needs should be comprehensive and tailored to a person's current and projected needs, taking into account patients' and carers' views.[8] The accurate and robust assessment of individual people's needs has been the focus of increasing discussion in clinical settings for older people with respect to an increasing ageing population. This debate arises from services negligence or the inability to meet older peoples' needs, which has resulted from age-discriminatory practices, failure to treat older people with dignity and respect, lack of best evidence-based clinical practice and allowing organisational structures to create barriers for receiving proper assessment of need and access to care.[4] Older people's needs and preferences must be carefully taken into consideration, and care plans should be designed to improve health outcomes and enhance the quality of their lives.

The inclusion of self-reported patient outcomes raises complex questions about accuracy, effectiveness and the experience for users. The ability to participate in needs assessments may be affected by the older person's physical and mental wellbeing, cognitive impairment and feelings of vulnerability, or the assessments may be burdensome to complete.[9] This can be countered by including older people's views in the development of scales with regard to format, relevance and mode of implementation.[10] While differences in the perceptions of needs may exist between older people and professionals, the person's subjective assessment should not be ignored because the professional disagrees. What is important is that the older person's perception has been communicated successfully in terms of their needs and that the assessment leads to improvement in care.[9] More importantly, the inclusion of the older person's views may allow for the identification of unmet needs that otherwise may have been missed, so professional assessments alone may not be adequate to determine the need for care.

1.3 Camberwell Assessment of Need for the Elderly

The Camberwell Assessment of Need for the Elderly (CANE)[11] is an instrument designed for measuring the broad range of needs in older people. It is designed to be used across various clinical and social care settings and is based on the structural model of the Camberwell Assessment of Need.[12] In 2004, a single publication providing comprehensive information about the CANE was produced in direct response to the growing demand for validated needs assessment in the United Kingdom and internationally.[8] The publication, written by contributors from different countries, showed the CANE's adaptability in terms of being used in various settings and for being translated into other languages. It included a manual for its use that contained the final version of the CANE instrument.

Twenty years on from the CANE's development, it is now time to look again at how it has been used and its relevance for older people's health services around the world. This second edition of the *Camberwell Assessment of Needs for the Elderly (CANE)* will include an overview and new perspectives on how the CANE has been used to assess the needs of older people across a range of settings internationally. This first chapter provides an overview of the evidence base for how the CANE has been established internationally and the clinical contexts in which it has been implemented.

1.4 Structure of the CANE

The instrument 'Camberwell Assessment of Needs in Elderly' was developed and designed by using the Delphi consensus method to gather information about older people's needs and identify whether they are being met or not.[11] This process included consultation with academics, practitioners, carers and older people's patient groups. The CANE comprises 24 items; it additionally

Table 1.1 Items Included in the Camberwell Assessment of Need for the Elderly

1. Accommodation
2. Looking after the home
3. Food
4. Self-care
5. Caring for someone else
6. Daytime activities
7. Memory
8. Eyesight/hearing
9. Mobility/falls
10. Continence
11. Physical health
12. Drugs
13. Psychotic symptoms
14. Psychological distress
15. Information (on condition and treatment)
16. Safety to self (deliberate self-harm)
17. Safety to self (inadvertent self-harm)
18. Safety to self (abuse/neglect)
19. Behaviour
20. Alcohol
21. Company
22. Intimate relationships
23. Money/budgeting
24. Benefits
A. Carers need for information
B. Carers psychological distress

has two items to assess carer needs (see Table 1.1). The instrument offers a multidimensional approach, with the items being constructed around four domains that cover physical, psychological, social and environmental needs. The nature and severity of difficulty in each domain are explored, as are the level of help received and the perceived need for help. A multi-agency perspective is also provided, as the CANE seeks staff, patients' and carers' views about an individual's needs. The inclusion of self-assessment is important as it allows the concerns of the person to be identified, which influences the care planning process and promotes individualised care.[9] The CANE has been used to assess the health and social needs of older populations in many countries across the world, as it is proven to be a good assessment tool with good psychometric properties that accurately and reliably assesses older people's individual needs, both met and unmet, from different perspectives.

1.5 International Use of the CANE

Since the publication of the first edition of the CANE book,[8] Martin Orrell, one of the editors, has maintained a database compiled of contacts requesting information about the tool or requesting permission to translate and use the CANE, either clinically or for service evaluation and research. Information from the CANE database shows requests to use the CANE in 33 countries worldwide (United Kingdom, United States, South America, Europe, Asia, South Africa and Middle East) and in 18 languages (English, Dutch, German, Polish, French, Spanish, Italian, Portuguese, Icelandic, Finnish, Norwegian, Turkish, Chinese, Japanese, Korean, Farsi, Hebrew and Hindi).

An internet search on needs assessment for older people found publications using translated versions of the CANE in 10 other languages (Dutch, German, Polish, Spanish, Portuguese, Norwegian, Arabic, Korean, Farsi and Thai), which have been used in research studies across 24 different countries (Australia, Brazil, Canada, Chile, China, Denmark, Finland, Germany, Netherlands, Iceland, Iran, Ireland, Italy, Korea, Lebanon, Malaysia, Norway, Poland, Portugal, Spain, Sweden, Thailand, United States and United Kingdom). Many of the studies were multisite studies (national or international) or studies that used adapted versions of the CANE.

1.6 Translations and Adaptations of the CANE

As the CANE has been translated into other languages, studies have been undertaken to test the validity and reliability of the translated versions. These studies have been undertaken across a diverse range of community and healthcare settings and applied to the general older population or specific patient groups, such as those with dementia or depression.

One of the first CANE translations was into the Spanish language, and this study was included as a chapter in the first CANE book.[13] Mateos et al.[14] undertook a further study to establish the validity of the Spanish version of the CANE. This study consisted of an epidemiological survey, where interviews were conducted in the homes of 800 older people by lay interviewers. The CANE was then self-completed by 365 older people and 66 carers. The CANE was found to be acceptable, easy to apply and have good concurrent validity compared with other instruments that measured psychiatric symptoms, dependence

and carer burden. The Spanish version of the CANE has been used subsequently in Chile to effectively assess the met and unmet needs of a community sample of 166 people with dementia and their family carers.[15]

A further translation of the CANE to Portuguese was undertaken by Gonçalves-Pereira et al.[16] and piloted with 21 older people, most of whom had dementia and lived at home with a carer. The CANE was found to have good acceptability, although there were concerns about its practical application clinically. Subsequently, Fernandes et al.[17] conducted a cross-sectional multicenter study with 79 participants who used mental health services in Portugal and evaluated the reliability and validity of the Portuguese version of the CANE. The study concluded that the Portuguese version of the CANE tool had excellent validity and reliability, with robust results for ecological, face, content, criterion and construct validity as well as for reliability. The Portuguese version of the CANE was viewed as potentially being useful for research and practical use in old age mental health services. Sousa et al.[18] also used the Portuguese version of the CANE to assess the feasibility of using the instrument to measure the needs of a disadvantaged older population in Brazil. The study was conducted as part of the São Paulo Ageing and Health Study and included a sample of 32 older people using community health services. The CANE was found to have robust psychometric properties and was feasible and practical for use to measure the needs of older people with limited access to health and social care. However, it was observed that the CANE took longer to administer than in higher-income countries given that participants had little formal education.

Elsewhere in Europe, translated versions of the CANE have continued to show good psychometric properties. The validity and reliability of the Dutch version of the CANE[19] were assessed using a sample of 236 people with mild to severe dementia and 322 informal carers living in the community.[20] The study showed acceptable construct and criterion validity. Test-retest reliability showed moderate to good levels of agreement, which was better on domains where needs were explicit, such as deliberate self-harm, self-care, drugs and continence, but poorer in areas where problems were less well defined, such as the areas for information and intimate relationships. In Poland, Rymaszewska et al.[21] assessed the validity, reliability and feasibility of using the Polish short version of the CANE. The sample included 70 older people receiving dialysis or rehabilitation, and the CANE was found to have good psychometric properties and acceptability for use within Polish healthcare. A study of the relevance and applicability of the German version of the CANE also was published in the first CANE book.[22] A further study to test the reliability of using the German version of the CANE was undertaken with 94 nursing home residents.[23] Psychometric testing showed acceptable levels of agreement, and the CANE was observed to be an effective instrument for assessing residents' needs. However, it was recommended that the short version of the CANE be used in nursing homes. Following on, a study was undertaken to assess the content validity of a modified version of the German CANE, in which the instrument was adapted for use within German healthcare settings.[24] The layout of the instrument was reformatted and additional instructions for its use added. Changes were made based on expert recommendations to the prompts used as examples for assessing needs, and extensions were added to existing domains to include dental health, disability, pain and delirium. The domain item 'alcohol' was amended to 'abuse and addiction', and a new section was added for falls. The revised German version of the CANE was perceived as being a more practical instrument with high content validity and increased applicability for use with the older population in Germany.

The CANE has also been translated into languages used in the Middle East. AliHabib et al.[25] assessed the feasibility, reliability and construct validity of the Arabic version of the CANE. It was used to investigate the post-war psychosocial needs and health of 322 older people living in South Lebanon. The Arabic version of the CANE was found to have good psychometric properties and acceptability within the predominantly Muslim population and was deemed to be an appropriate and useful tool for Middle Eastern community settings. Similarly, the Persian version of the CANE was used to assess the needs of 123 older people with mental health problems and their carers in Iran[26] and was also found to demonstrate good validity, reliability and acceptability within this population.

Additional translations have been undertaken in Asia, which also showed good psychometric properties. The Thai version of the CANE was used to effectively assess the needs of 330 older people living in the community.[27] Parks et al.[28] tested the Korean version

of the CANE with 359 family carers of people with dementia. The CANE-K was well accepted and could accurately identify the needs of participants. It was seen as providing a useful basis for person-centred care planning and creating a care framework for people with dementia. In China, the content and methods for administering the CANE were used to inform the development of an interview guide to assess the healthcare, physical, security and financial, psychological, social and spiritual needs of older people.[29]

The English version of the CANE has also been used in Malaysia and India, where English is commonly used to bridge the diversity of spoken languages in healthcare. Ashokkumar et al.[30] identified the health and social care needs in a rural community sample of 305 older people in India. The commonest unmet needs were lack of age-appropriate accommodation, company and daytime activities, with difficulty in looking after the home and risk of abuse and neglect also being commonplace. Recommendations were made for a more targeted approach to identify at-risk older people living in rural communities and to provide services to reduce the burden of unmet need. The short version of the CANE was used to assess the needs of 110 care home residents with dementia in Malaysia.[31] The commonest unmet needs identified were for daytime activity, company and intimate relationships, with social isolation being the strongest predictor for unmet needs in this population.

1.7 Adaptations of the CANE

Iliffe et al.[32] developed a shorter needs assessment tool for use in routine primary care. Data from 544 CANE interviews undertaken with older people in primary care, day hospital and continuing care settings were analysed to identify and rank the commonest unmet needs. Following a process of consultation and consensus, five domains of unmet need were identified as priority areas to create the SPICE assessment tool.[33] The five areas were *S*enses (vision and hearing), *P*hysical ability (mobility and falls), *I*ncontinence, *C*ognition and *E*motional distress (depression and anxiety) (SPICE). The SPICE tool was subsequently translated into a Portuguese version[34] and used to assess the needs of 51 older people attending general practitioner (GP) practices in Portugal. The tool was found to be acceptable to both patients and GPs, but only a few GPs planned to use it further clinically because of time constraints.

Murray et al.[35] developed and tested a primary care–based model for stroke aftercare. The aim of the model was to meet the longer-term needs of people who have had a stroke. In developing the model, common problem areas related to physical, psychological, social and environmental aspects were mapped to items within the available needs assessments tools including the CANE, EASY-Care[36] and the Minimum Data Set for Home Care (MDS-HC).[37] The CANE was identified as providing the best selection of questions for the problem areas identified, but none fully matched the problem areas identified, so a selection of questions was used from the CANE and EASY-Care.[38] The needs assessment tools were considered administratively cumbersome, and there were concerns that they may be burdensome for patients to complete. However, the model was acceptable to the health and social care practitioners administering the tool and found to be useful for identifying unmet needs that informed the care planning process.

The Dutch version of the CANE was incorporated into the Geriatric Care Model[39] to assess the care needs of 1,147 frail older people in 35 primary care practices in the Netherlands.[40] The Geriatric Care Model consisted of multidimensional geriatric assessments undertaken every six months by practice nurses to identify care interventions and formulate care plans to improve health outcomes. However, evaluation of the Geriatric Care Model approach showed no significant benefits for improving the quality of life or health outcomes of the frail older population in comparison to those receiving usual care. The study posited that comprehensive care programmes may have little effect where high-quality healthcare services are already meeting the needs of the population.

1.8 Needs Assessment and Community Health

The availability of the CANE in several languages makes it a valuable tool for identifying and comparing the needs of older people globally. While the CANE instrument was designed primarily for use with older people with mental health needs, its application is not necessarily restricted to this population. As observed in the preceding section, different versions of the CANE were validated for use with older people across a range of specific public health and mental health settings, including care homes.

Research has been undertaken in several additional community-based studies to identify the met and unmet needs of the general older population or specific patient groups. Walters et al.[41] used the CANE to explore help-seeking behaviour in older people attending four London GP practices. More than three-quarters of the 55 patients and 15 carers assessed had not sought help for the unmet needs identified, which mostly related to physical, psychological and accommodation needs such as continence and mobility issues, depressive symptoms and the need for adaptations in the home. Barriers were perceived as being due to low motivation to seek help and low expectations of the help that was available. Similarly, Stein et al.[42] used the original German version of the CANE to assess the needs of older patients from GP practices in Germany and found that many had unmet needs. The mean age of the sample was 80 years, and the most commonly identified unmet needs reported were in the physical domain (for physical health, eyesight/hearing/communication, mobility/falls and continence) and the environmental domain (for looking after the home and food). The physical and environmental domains had the highest number of overall needs, whereas the highest number of unmet care needs were found in the psychosocial domain, particularly for company. It was concluded that more attention should be paid to the psychosocial needs of frail older adults. Likewise, in the Netherlands, the assessment of self-perceived met and unmet needs in a community sample of 1,137 frail older people found that the highest number of care needs were in the physical and environmental domains, which were mostly met.[43] The highest proportions of unmet needs were found in the psychosocial domain for company and daytime activities and were associated with age, dependency and frailty scores. An additional study undertaken in the Netherlands explored the self-perceived needs of 407 frail older people with joint pain and co-morbidity.[44] High numbers of needs were reported in the environmental and physical domains using the CANE, but most of these needs were met. Whereas fewer needs were reported in the psychological domain, living alone and perceptions of low social support were associated with more unmet needs for company and daytime activities.

A survey incorporating questions from the CANE was used to assess the needs of an older homeless population in Canada.[45] The survey was completed by homeless shelter managers and identified increased prevalence of memory impairment, verbal aggression and alcohol abuse in older men and memory impairment, paranoia and depression in older women. Unmet needs were associated with memory difficulties, concurrent physical illness, restricted mobility and difficulty with self-care. The need for a more comprehensive approach to assessing and treating the homeless older population was advocated, with greater involvement being required from psychiatric services.

1.9 Needs Assessment and Mental Health

The CANE has also been used to specifically assess the mental health needs of older populations in primary, secondary and care home settings. Passos et al.[46] assessed the needs of 306 older people attending outpatient and inpatient mental health services in Portugal, which included people diagnosed with depression, dementia and schizophrenia. The most common unmet needs for patients were psychological distress, daytime activities and benefits, although there was disparity among staff, patient and carer ratings. People with dementia and those who were inpatients were found to have the greatest number of needs, whereas those with depression had the least. Other studies undertaken in Europe and Australia have found that people with dementia in community and care home settings have higher-rated needs across all the domains than those without dementia, and self-ratings tend to be lower than those of carers and staff.[47–51] Community samples of people with depression in Germany were also found to have higher numbers of rated unmet needs than those without.[52] The commonest unmet needs reported were for physical health, mobility/falls, company, psychological distress and daytime activities. Similarly, people with depression in the Netherlands rated unmet needs for daytime activities, intimate relationships, eyesight/hearing and company, and higher levels of unmet need were associated with higher levels of depression severity.[53] Care for people with depression is mainly provided in the psychological domain, and satisfaction is lowest for social care needs.[54] Patients with depression were also observed to score more unmet needs than staff and carers, which may be due to staff and carers' lack of awareness about patient's unmet need.[55]

The needs of older people diagnosed with severe mental illness (major depressive illness, schizophrenia and bipolar disorder) using adult and old age mental health services were assessed in the United Kingdom,[56] Netherlands,[57,58] Australia[59] and the United States.[60] The studies found generally good agreement between patients and staff for the number of needs reported, with needs reported in the psychological, physical and environmental domains being mostly met. This is mainly due to patients living within residential or supportive accommodation.[56] The highest number of unmet needs was consistently reported in the social domain for company and daytime activities and intimate relationships, which were linked to a lower quality of life and lack of social participation[58] or where the person was living alone.[60] It was noted that people with bipolar disorder reported a lower number of met and unmet needs than those with depression and schizophrenia.[58] Cummings and Klopf[61] found that although services provided care to meet the older person's need, for 70% of the US participants, this was not the right type of help for some needs, such as benefits and social contact, and identified the need for better integration with older people's services.

1.10 Conclusion

The CANE has been widely translated and validated for use in a variety of locations, including community, inpatient and care home setting. The versatility of the CANE instrument is evident in the breadth of studies in which it has been successfully applied to effectively assess the needs of older populations with a range of health needs. It provides a comprehensive and structured assessment that can be used by different health and social care professionals to consistently identify both the met and unmet needs of older people.

High numbers of unmet need continue to be identified within older people's populations that identify gaps in service provision. As health services adapt to meet the needs of a growing older population, it is important that future research evaluates the impact of these changes on older people's needs and health outcomes. Failure to meet the unmet needs of older people can result in poorer quality of life and ineffective use of resources and lead to a substantial increase in costs to health and social care services. This second edition of the *Camberwell Assessment of Needs for the Elderly (CANE)* will examine the needs of older people further and identify where areas of care can be improved. Most of the chapters focus on the needs of people living with dementia, and this reflects the global healthcare priority for research and needs assessment in dementia.[62] This second edition provides a valuable addition to the expanding collection of international needs assessment research in older people.

References

1. Wright J, Williams R, Wilkinson JR. Development and importance of health needs assessment. *British Medical Journal* 1998; **316**(7140):1310–13.

2. Stevens A, Raftery J, Mant J, Simpson S. *Health Care Needs Assessment: The Epidemiologically Based Needs Assessment Reviews*. London: Radcliffe Publishing; 2004.

3. Hensher M, Fulop N. The influence of health needs assessment on health care decision-making in London health authorities. *Journal of Health Services Research & Policy* 1999; **4**(2):90–5.

4. Department of Health (DoH). *National Service Framework for Older People*. London: Department of Health; 2001.

5. Oliver D, Foot C, Humphries R. *Making Our Health and Care Systems Fit for an Ageing Population*. London: King's Fund; 2014.

6. Ham C, Dixon A, Brooke B. *Transforming the Delivery of Health and Social Care*. London: King's Fund; 2012.

7. United Nations. *World Population Ageing 2017: Highlights*. New York: UN Department of Economic and Social Affairs; 2017.

8. Orrell M, Hancock G, eds. *CANE – Camberwell Assessment of Need for the Elderly: A Needs Assessment for Older Mental Health Service Users*. London: Gaskell; 2004.

9. Griffiths P, Ullman V, Harris R. Self-assessment of health and social care needs by older people: A multi-method systematic review of practices, accuracy, effectiveness and experience. London: National Co-ordinating Centre for NHS Service Delivery and Organisation; 2005.

10. Haywood KL, Garratt A, Schmidt L, Mackintosh A, Fitzpatrick R. *Health Status and Quality of Life in Older People: A Structured Review of Patient-Reported Health Instruments*. Oxford: Oxford University Press; 2004.

11. Reynolds T, Thornicroft G, Abas M, et al. Camberwell Assessment of Need for the Elderly (CANE): Development, validity and reliability. *British Journal of Psychiatry* 2000; **176**(5):444–52.

12. Phelan M, Slade M, Thornicroft G, et al. The Camberwell Assessment of Need: The validity and reliability of an instrument to assess the needs of people with severe mental illness. *British Journal of Psychiatry* 1995; **167**(5):589–95.

13. Mateos R, Ybarzábal M, Garcia M, et al. The Spanish CANE: Validation study and utility in epidemiological surveys. In Orrell M, Hancock G (eds.), *CANE: Camberwell Assessment of Need for the Elderly*. London: Gaskell; 2004:21–8.

14. Mateos R, Ybarzábal M, Amboage MT, Crespo JM. The suitability of the Camberwell Assessment of Needs of the Elderly in epidemiological surveys: Further evidence on the validity of the Spanish version of CANE. Poster presentation at the Instrument for Pre-Accession Assistance (IPA) European Regional Meeting, Brussels; 2003.

15. Muñoz TT, Slachevsky A, León-Campos MO, et al. Predictors of unmet needs in Chilean older people with dementia: A cross-sectional study. *BMC Geriatrics* 2019; **19**(1):1–10.

16. Gonçalves-Pereira M, Fernandes L, Leuschner A, et al. Versão portuguesa do CANE (Camberwell Assessment of Need for the Elderly): Desenvolvimento e dados preliminares. *Revista Portuguesa de Saúde Pública* 2007; **25**(1):7–18.

17. Fernandes L, Gonçalves-Pereira M, Leuschner A, et al. Validation study of the Camberwell Assessment of Need for the Elderly (CANE) in Portugal. *International Psychogeriatrics* 2009; **21**(1):94.

18. Sousa RM, Scazufca M, Menezes PR, Crepaldi AL, Prince MJ. Feasibility and reliability of the elderly version of the Camberwell Assessment of Needs (CANE): Results from the Sao Paulo Ageing & Health Study. *Brazilian Journal of Psychiatry* 2009; **31**(1):34–8.

19. Dröes RM, Van Hout HP, van der Ploeg ES. *Camberwell Assessment of Need for the Elderly (CANE)*, revised version (IV). Amsterdam: EMGO Institute; 2004.

20. van der Roest HG, Meiland FJ, van Hout HP, Jonker C, Dröes RM. Validity and reliability of the Dutch version of the Camberwell Assessment of Need for the Elderly in community-dwelling people with dementia. *International Psychogeriatrics* 2008; **20**(6):1273–90.

21. Rymaszewska J, Kłak R, Synak A. Camberwell Assessment of Need for the Elderly (CANE): Badanie polskiej wersji narzędzia. *Psychogeriatria Polska* 2008; **5**(2):105–13.

22. Dech H, Machleidt W. Relevance and applicability of the CANE in the German health care system. In Orrell M, Hancock G. (eds.), *CANE: Camberwell Assessment of Need for the Elderly*. London: Gaskell; 2004:29–34.

23. Fink HA. Testing of the Camberwell Assessment of Need for the Elderly (CANE) in a German setting. Unpublished PhD dissertation, University of Berlin, Berlin, Germany; 2011.

24. Stein J, Luppa M, König HH, Riedel-Heller SG. The German version of the Camberwell Assessment of Need for the Elderly (CANE): Evaluation of content validity and adaptation to the German-speaking context. *International Psychogeriatrics* 2015; **27**(11):1919–26.

25. AbiHabib LE, Chemaitelly HS, Jaalouk LY, Karam NE. Developing capacities in aging studies in the Middle East: Implementation of an Arabic version of the CANE IV among community-dwelling older adults in Lebanon. *Aging & Mental Health* 2011; **15**(5):605–17.

26. Salehi R, Davatgaran K, Heidari M, Mostafaee N, Latifi M. The psychometric properties of the Persian version of the Camberwell Assessment of Needs (CANE) for Iranian elderly people with mental disorders. *Iranian Journal of Ageing* 2018; **13**(2):168–81.

27. Tiativiriyakul P, Xenos P. Assessment of need for elderly in community in Hang Dong District, Chiang Mai Province, Thailand using Camberwell Assessment of Need for the Elderly Questionnaire (CANE). *Journal of Health Research* 2017; **31**(Suppl. 2):S143–154.

28. Park M, Kim SK, Jeong M, et al. Psychometric validation of the Korean version of the Camberwell Assessment of Need for the Elderly in individuals with dementia. *Asian Nursing Research* 2018; **12**(2):106–12.

29. Chen H, Levkoff S. Assessing needs among elders in urban China: Interview and limitations. *Ageing International* 2017; **42**(2):159–68.

30. Ashokkumar T, Chacko TV, Munuswamy S. Health care and social needs of the elderly: Assessed by the tool Camberwell Assessment of Need for the Elderly. *International Journal of Tropical Medicine* 2011; **6**:97–9.

31. Nikmat AW, Almashoor SH. Older adults with cognitive impairment living in Malaysian nursing homes: Have we met their needs? *ASEAN Journal of Psychiatry* 2015; **16**(1):84–94.

32. Iliffe S, Lenihan P, Orrell M, et al. The development of a short instrument to identify common unmet needs in older people in general practice. *British Journal of General Practice* 2004; **54**(509):914–18.

33. Drennan V, Walters K, Lenihan P, et al. Priorities in identifying unmet need in older people attending general practice: A nominal group technique study. *Family Practice* 2007; **24**(5):454–60.

34. Balsinha C, Marques MJ, Gonçalves-Pereira M. A brief assessment unravels unmet needs of older people in primary care: A mixed-methods evaluation of the SPICE tool in Portugal. *Primary Health Care Research & Development* 2018; **19**(6):637–43.

35. Murray J, Young J, Forster A, Herbert G, Ashworth R. Feasibility study of a primary care-based model for stroke aftercare. *British Journal of General Practice* 2006; **56**(531):775–80.

36. Philp I. EASY-Care: A systematic approach to the assessment of older people. *Geriatric Medicine* 2000; **30**(5):15–19.

37. Carpenter GI. *InterRAI UK MDS Home Care Assessment Instrument for Community Care: User's Manual.* Kent, UK: University of Kent; 2002.

38. Murray J, Young J, Forster A. Review of longer-term problems after a disabling stroke. *Reviews in Clinical Gerontology* 2007; **17**(4):277–92.

39. Muntinga ME, Hoogendijk EO, Van Leeuwen KM, et al. Implementing the chronic care model for frail older adults in the Netherlands: Study protocol of ACT (frail older adults: care in transition). *BMC Geriatrics* 2012; **12**(1):1–10.

40. Hoogendijk EO, van der Horst HE, van de Ven PM, et al. Effectiveness of a geriatric care model for frail older adults in primary care: Results from a stepped wedge cluster randomized trial. *European Journal of Internal Medicine* 2016; **28**:43–51.

41. Walters K, Iliffe S, Orrell M. An exploration of help-seeking behaviour in older people with unmet needs. *Family Practice* 2001; **18**(3):277–82.

42. Stein J, Luppa M, König HH, Riedel-Heller SG. Assessing met and unmet needs in the oldest-old and psychometric properties of the German version of the Camberwell Assessment of Need for the Elderly (CANE): A pilot study. *International Psychogeriatrics* 2014; **26**(2):1–11.

43. Hoogendijk EO, Muntinga ME, van Leeuwen KM, et al. Self-perceived met and unmet care needs of frail older adults in primary care. *Archives of Gerontology and Geriatrics* 2014; **58**(1):37–42.

44. Hermsen LA, Hoogendijk EO, van der Wouden JC, et al. Self-perceived care needs in older adults with joint pain and comorbidity. *Aging Clinical and Experimental Research* 2018; **30**(5):449–55.

45. Stergiopoulos V, Herrmann N. Old and homeless: A review and survey of older adults who use shelters in an urban setting. *Canadian Journal of Psychiatry* 2003; **48**(6):374–80.

46. Passos J, Sequeira C, Fernandes L. The needs of older people with mental health problems: A particular focus on dementia patients and their carers. *International Journal of Alzheimer's Disease* 2012; 2012, https://doi.org/10.1155/2012/638267.

47. Stein J, Pabst A, Luck T, et al. Unmet care needs in the oldest old primary care patients with cognitive disorders: Results of the AgeCoDe and AgeQualiDe

study. *Dementia and Geriatric Cognitive Disorders* 2017; **44**(1–2):71–83.

48. Hopper L, Joyce R, Jelley H, et al. (Un)Met needs of community dwelling people with dementia: The importance of providing integrated holistic care. Presented at the 17th International Conference on Integrated Care, Dublin, Ireland, 8–10 May 2017.

49. van der Ploeg ES, Bax D, Boorsma M, Nijpels G, van Hout HP. A cross-sectional study to compare care needs of individuals with and without dementia in residential homes in the Netherlands. *BMC Geriatrics* 2013; **13**(1):1–8.

50. Wieczorowska-Tobis K, Talarska D, Kropińska S, et al. The Camberwell Assessment of Need for the Elderly questionnaire as a tool for the assessment of needs in elderly individuals living in long-term care institutions. *Archives of Gerontology and Geriatrics* 2016; **62**:163–8.

51. Ferreira AR, Dias CC, Fernandes L. Needs in nursing homes and their relation with cognitive and functional decline, behavioral and psychological symptoms. *Frontiers in Aging Neuroscience* 2016; **8**:1–10.

52. Stein J, Pabst A, Weyerer S, et al. The assessment of met and unmet care needs in the oldest old with and without depression using the Camberwell Assessment of Need for the Elderly (CANE): Results of the AgeMooDe study. *Journal of Affective Disorders* 2016; **193**:309–17.

53. Houtjes W, Van Meijel B, Deeg DJ, Beekman AT. Major depressive disorder in late life: A multifocus perspective on care needs. *Aging & Mental Health* 2010; **14**(7):874–80.

54. Clignet F, Houtjes W, van Straten A, Cuijpers P, van Meijel B. Unmet care needs, care provision and

patient satisfaction in patients with a late life depression: A cross-sectional study. *Aging & Mental Health* 2019; **23**(4):491–7.

55. Houtjes W, van Meijel B, Deeg DJ, Beekman AT. Unmet needs of outpatients with late-life depression: A comparison of patient, staff and carer perceptions. *Journal of Affective Disorders* 2011; **134**(1–3):242–8.

56. Sultan S, Claassen D, Stansfeld S. Older people with long-term mental illness: A survey in a community rehabilitation service using the Camberwell Assessment of Needs for the Elderly (CANE). *British Journal of Medical Practitioners* 2011; **4**(4):22–5.

57. Meesters PD, Comijs HC, Droes RM, et al. The care needs of elderly patients with schizophrenia spectrum disorders. *American Journal of Geriatric Psychiatry* 2013; **21**(2):129–37.

58. Dautzenberg G, Lans L, Meesters PD, et al. The care needs of older patients with bipolar disorder. *Aging & Mental Health* 2016; **20**(9):899–907.

59. Futeran S, Draper BM. An examination of the needs of older patients with chronic mental illness in public mental health services. *Aging & Mental Health* 2012; **16**(3):327–34.

60. Cummings SM, Cassie KM. Perceptions of biopsychosocial services needs among older adults with severe mental illness: Met and unmet needs. *Health & Social Work* 2008; **33**(2):133–43.

61. Cummings SM, Kropf NP. Formal and informal support for older adults with severe mental illness. *Aging & Mental Health* 2009; **13**(4):619–27.

62. World Health Organization. *Global Action Plan on the Public Health Response to Dementia, 2017–2025*. Geneva: WHO; 2018:20.

Chapter 2

Self-Reported Needs of People with Dementia Living at Home
A Scoping Review

Alžběta Bártová, Iva Holmerová, Vladimíra Dostálová, Hana Bláhová and Michal Šteffl

2.1 Introduction

Demographic changes are associated with an increased number of people with dementia.[1] Cognitive communication disorders and reduced ability to use the environment to meet one's own needs are part of the dementia syndrome.[2] The relationship between meeting one´s needs and quality of life is generally accepted.[3] Quality of life is a very broad concept with different dimensions which can be approached from many perspectives. Also, needs can be approached from different perspectives: for example, objective and subjective.[4] Objective needs can be measured by relevant tools or reported by family or professional carers,[5] whereas subjective needs are based on individual feelings and self-perception.[6,7] Previous studies have shown that a higher quality of life is related to a lower number of unmet needs.[6,8,9] To ensure an adequate quality of life for a person with dementia, it is necessary to focus on meeting their objective as well as subjective needs.

Understanding and meeting the needs of people with dementia are particularly problematic because of dementia symptoms, for example, changed comprehension and difficulties in communication. However, the care experiences of people with dementia bring meaningful and useful information about their needs.[10] Identifying the individual needs of a person with dementia is essential to ensure person-centred care[5,11] and to avoid or delay institutionalisation.[11]

There is an increasing amount of research that focuses on meeting the needs of people with dementia. However, most of this research is carried out in residential establishments. Available research on the needs of people with dementia living in their home environment focuses mostly on the carers' perspective, and some studies focus directly on carers' needs.[12] Although family carers play an important role in identifying and addressing the unmet needs of care recipients,[13] people with dementia are important informants about their own life and subjective well-being.[14,15] Previous studies have pointed out that people with dementia typically report a significantly lower number of unmet needs than their carers.[7–9,16,17] Even though differences between perspectives confirm the importance of examining the self-reported needs of people with dementia,[9] there is a lack of studies evaluating the subjective needs of people with dementia.[5,12,18] The aim of this scoping review therefore is to provide an overview of the self-reported needs of home-dwelling people with dementia.

2.2 Method

2.2.1 Scoping Review Methodology

In order to provide an overview of this area and because of the lack of current research, a scoping review was selected as the appropriate methodology for this study. A scoping review maps the nature and extent of research and determines gaps in research activity to direct future research.[19] The scoping review methodology is described as a six-stage framework: (1) identifying the research question, (2) searching for relevant studies, (3) selecting studies, (4) charting the data, (5) collating, summarising and reporting the results and (6) consulting with stakeholders to inform or validate study findings.[20] Recommendations to clarify and enhance each stage[21] were used for the purposes of this review.

2.2.2 Search Strategy

The databases PubMed, Web of Science, PsycINFO and Scopus were used in the search, which took place during August and September 2019. The search was initially narrowed to include articles published between January 2009 and August 2019 in English or Czech using search terms 'dementia' and 'needs', which resulted in a total of 814 articles, and 18 articles were identified through other sources.

2.2.3 Inclusion and Exclusion Criteria

The inclusion and exclusion criteria were decided upon through discussion by authors AB, VD and IH and were reviewed by all authors throughout the process. Articles of both quantitative and qualitative study designs were included. After discarding duplicates, the authors identified appropriate studies using the primary inclusion criteria, that is, exploring the needs of people with dementia. Articles that examined the needs of people with dementia in a hospital or a long-term care facility were excluded from the review. Studies not seeking to obtain views of people with dementia themselves were not included. To ensure the quality and transparency of the screening process, the Preferred Reporting Items for Systematic Reviews and Meta-Analyses (PRISMA) recommendation for systematic evaluation was carried out (Figure 2.1).

2.3 Results

2.3.1 Study Characteristics

The final review includes 13 studies both quantitative ($n = 11$) and qualitative ($n = 2$). Most of the quantitative studies were cross-sectional ($n = 8$); fewer were longitudinal ($n = 3$). As a measurement tool, the Camberwell Assessment of Needs for the Elderly (CANE) was used in most quantitative studies ($n = 7$), then the Johns Hopkins Dementia Care Needs Assessment (JHDCNA) was used in three quantitative studies, and finally, the DelpHi Standard was used in one study. Semi-structured and narrative interviews were used in qualitative studies. In addition to people with dementia, family caregivers (whose responses and results are not included in the survey) participated in most studies ($n = 12$). All selected studies focused on people with dementia living in the community. Table 2.1 provides a summary of the individual studies.

2.3.2 Domains of Reported Needs

Clear division of needs is difficult.[22] In the available studies included in this scoping review, the

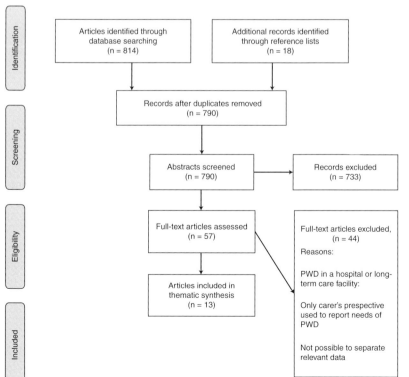

Figure 2.1 Search flowchart in accordance with PRISMA guidelines

Identification

| Articles identified through database searching (n = 814) | Additional records identified through reference lists (n = 18) |

Screening

Records after duplicates removed (n = 790)

Abstracts screened (n = 790) → Records excluded (n = 733)

Eligibility

Full-text articles assessed (n = 57) → Full-text articles excluded, (n = 44)

Reasons:

PWD in a hospital or long-term care facility:

Only carer's prespective used to report needs of PWD

Not possible to separate relevant data

Included

Articles included in thematic synthesis (n = 13)

Table 2.1 Summary of Articles Used in Thematic Analysis

Author (Year)/ Country	Aim	Study Population	Research Type	Assessments/ Tools	Reported Needs
Black et al. (2013)/USA	To determine the prevalence and correlates of unmet needs in a sample of community-residing people with dementia and their family caregivers	Community-residing persons with dementia (n = 254) and their family caregivers (n = 246)	Quantitative	JHDCNA	Safety: • Fall risk management • Home safety evaluation • Wander risk management General health and medical care Meaningful activities Legal issues and advance care planning Evaluation and diagnosis of dementia
Black et al. (2019)/USA	Determine the percentage of people with dementia having unmet needs and significant correlates of unmet needs in people with dementia	Community-living people with dementia and their family caregivers (n = 646)	Quantitative	JHDCNA	Home/personal safety • Need for emergency planning • Fall risk management • Medication use General healthcare Daily activities Neuropsychiatric symptoms management Legal issues and advance care planning
Eichler et al. (2016)/ Germany	To describe the number and types of unmet needs of German primary care patients screened positive for dementia and factors associated with the number of unmet needs	227 persons with dementia (≥70 years, living at home) of the intervention group who had screened positive for dementia	Quantitative	DelpHi Standard of Optimum Care	Social counselling and legal support mainly in power of attorney/legal representative Social integration/physical activities Pharmaceutical treatment and care Mobility limitation/risk of fall
Górska et al. (2013)/UK	This study aimed to develop a deeper understanding of the lived experience of people with dementia regarding their service-related needs	31 participants: 12 persons with dementia (39%) and 19 unpaid carers (61%)	Qualitative	Semi-structured, narrative interviews	• Diagnostic services • Post-diagnostic support • Coordination • Continuity • Non-pharmacological intervention
Johnston et al. (2011)/ USA	Determine whether a telephone screening method could identify individuals in the community in need of care for dementia; develop a multidimensional needs assessment tool for identifying the unmet needs related to memory disorders in the home setting	13 persons with dementia and carers	Quantitative	JHDCNA	Need for a dementia workup General medical care Environmental safety Assistance with activities of daily living impairments Access to meaningful activities

Study/Country	Aim	Design	Instrument	Sample	Needs/domains
Kerpershoek et al. (2017)/INT	To describe the domains and level of needs in a group of people with dementia and their family carers who do not yet use formal care and to describe the relationship of needs and quality of life from different perspectives	Quantitative	CANE	451 community-dwelling people with dementia and their carers participated from eight European countries	Company Information Daytime activities
Mazurek et al. (2017)/Poland	Assess the needs of people with dementia living at home	Quantitative	CANE	47 people diagnosed with mild to moderate dementia and 41 family carers	Psychological distress Company Daytime activities
Mazurek et al. (2019)/Poland	Investigate whether the Meeting Centres Support Programme (MCSP) is effective in meeting the needs of older people with dementia	Quantitative	CANE	47 people diagnosed with mild to moderate dementia and 42 family carers	Daytime activities Psychological distress Company Memory
Miranda-Castillo et al. (2010)/UK	Identify the relationship between unmet needs, social networks and quality of life of people with dementia living at home	Quantitative	CANE	152 community-dwelling people with dementia and 128 carers	Daytime activities Company Psychological distress Eyesight/hearing Accidental self-harm
Miranda-Castillo et al. (2010)/UK	Identify the needs of people with dementia living alone and to compare the needs of people with dementia living alone versus those living with others	Quantitative	CANE	Of 152 people with dementia, one-third of the people with dementia (n = 50) were living alone and 128 carers	Daytime activities Company Psychological distress Eyesight/hearing Accidental self-harm
Miranda-Castillo et al. (2013)/UK	Compare perspectives on perceived needs among community-residing people with dementia, their family caregivers and professionals	Quantitative	CANE	125 community-dwelling people with dementia and carers	Psychological distress Daytime activities Company Information Eyesight/hearing
Morrisby et al. (2018)/Australia	To identify care and support needs, as reported by people with dementia and their spousal carers living in the community in metropolitan western Australia	Qualitative	Semi-structured interviews	10 dyads of spousal carers and people with dementia	Environmental enablers to support care Adaptation of daily life roles
van der Roest et al. (2009)/Netherlands	Assess the needs of community-dwelling people with dementia as reported by themselves and by their family carers; provide insight into the service use and gaps between needs and the availability of services	Quantitative	CANE	236 community-dwelling people with dementia and 322 family carers interviewed separately	Memory Information Company Psychological distress Daytime activities

communicated needs are categorised either through domains of individual questionnaires or by placing them in hierarchical needs models. However, the categories overlap, and the sorting is not exact. Needs interact with each other when an unmet need in one area causes an unmet need in another area.[14]

Each of the three assessments used in quantitative research contains different domains and numbers of items. Therefore, differences in unmet needs are reported in terms of using different assessments as well as needs reported in qualitative studies. A total of seven most frequently reported needs were identified according to the CANE assessment: information, company, daytime activities, psychological distress, memory, eyesight/hearing and accidental self-harm. Six most commonly mentioned needs were identified using the JHDCNA in the following areas: dementia evaluation or diagnosis, dementia workup, legal issues and advance care planning, meaningful/daily activities, general health and medical care and safety home and personal. DelpHi Standard of Optimum Care shows unmet needs in the following domains: social counselling and legal support mainly in power of attorney/legal representative, the need to increase physical activities listed in domain of social integration, pharmaceutical treatment and care and nursing treatment and care, especially in case of mobility limitation/risk of fall. In qualitative studies, people with dementia identified their unmet needs in the following areas: diagnosis, post-diagnostic care, environmental support, meaningful activities and roles and safe home and community.

To achieve the aim of the scoping review, a thematic analysis was chosen to unify reported needs. For thematic analyses, the constant comparative method has been used,[23] which revealed a total of five themes specified by subthemes: environmental needs (dementia evaluation or diagnosis, post-diagnostic support), social needs (company, meaningful activities and roles), psychological needs (psychological distress, memory), biological/physical needs (general physical health) and need of safety (home, personal and environmental).

2.3.3 Environmental Needs: Expert Services and Environmental Enabling Factors

2.3.3.1 Dementia Evaluation or Diagnosis

Timely diagnosis was seen as an essential factor to access optimal services and drugs. Delayed diagnosis

has often been associated with lost opportunities to better manage the condition.[24] In one study, almost one-third of the people with dementia did not get prior dementia evaluation or diagnosis.[25] Numerous obstacles have been identified in obtaining a diagnosis, mainly due to inappropriate attitudes of primary care physicians. In some cases, especially when concerns were raised in the very early stages of dementia, it was reported that study participants[24] were advised to treat their symptoms as signs of normal ageing. Lack of communication between the services involved (primary care and specialised services) was cited as another possible cause of a delayed diagnosis. Insufficient coordination of the services forces people with dementia or their carers to secure medical examinations and transfer of information between services.[24] Many people with dementia identified unmet needs in the post-diagnostic phase: during the process from diagnosis to ongoing care. They experienced a lack of empathy from healthcare professionals and inconsistency of care provided (e.g., lack of referral to support services).[18]

2.3.3.2 Post-Diagnostic Support

Information and Coordination. People with dementia highly appreciate the continuous communication and information about their condition from diagnosis to referral to other available services. Better provision of information can help people with dementia to more accurately consider their needs; it also helps them to cope better with disease and to better use available services.[17] The need for access to information at one single place and coordination of available services have been identified as important for effective case management.[24] The need for information was reported by people with dementia as one of the most frequent unmet needs in a total of three studies.[7,8,17] The people directly reported that they either did not receive information at all or the received information was scarce or unclear (e.g., only printed without further explanation).[17] One study even stated that the area dementia workup was the most frequent (9/11) unmet need.[26] Information should be specifically adapted to individual needs and wishes and must be appropriate to the stage of the disease. The fact that people with dementia are experiencing the need for access to information should raise concerns in the current healthcare system and requires more attention.[26]

Continuity. Optimal care and access to quality services that meet the individual needs of people with dementia often result in strong and lasting relationships with service providers.[18] Continuity of care and especially appropriate involvement of health and welfare professionals were considered necessary for the provision of quality care.[24] People with dementia may have difficulties in recognising and remembering new people; they need enough time to develop a positive relationship. Discontinuity of services and frequent changes of service providers may cause increased anxiety for a person with dementia. While ensuring continuity of care services for people with dementia, service providers must also support their sense of confidentiality and security.[24]

Access to Non-Pharmacological Interventions/Psychosocial Interventions. The need for accessibility and availability of non-pharmacological interventions is also important. These interventions support identity and social participation and mitigate changes in physical and mental health. Prevention of reduced activity and interest has been highlighted as an essential element of high-quality care.[24]

Legal Issues and Advance Care Planning. The area of legal issues and advance care planning includes different items: choosing a person who will ensure the general and medical power of attorney for a person with dementia, documenting the last wishes and overseeing the estate.[11,25] Timely planning of these issues needs to be addressed well in advance while a person with dementia has decision-making capacity.[13] Social counselling and legal support were reported mainly in the area of power of attorney/legal representative.[11]

2.3.4 Social Needs

Social needs are among the most frequently mentioned needs in 12 of 13 studies. The most frequently mentioned themes in this domain are company[6–9,16,27] and meaningful daytime activities,[6–9,13,16,17,25,27] which are any activities that enable a person with dementia to engage in appropriate social, stimulating or leisure activities.[17] Losing meaningful activities and relationships, being useful for others or intimacy with a partner and the potential conflicts with relatives were specific situations that persons with dementia have listed under the item daytime activities and company.[17] Social integration,[11] everyday activities (e.g., household) and social roles (e.g., active grandparent role) are needed to maintain feelings of self-worth. Maintaining and continuing important roles or developing new roles requires the support of carers and sometimes also support services.[18] More than half of people with dementia reported unmet needs for meaningful activities that were described as day-care needs, visiting centres and home activities.[25] Unmet needs in daytime activities also include the need for help and support in the activities of daily living (ADLs), lack of meaningful activity or daily structure and physical inactivity or social isolation.[6] A supportive and knowledgeable social environment is also an important social need. The need for social support has three levels: family, friends and wider social networks.[18]

2.3.5 Psychological Needs: Mental State, Cognitive Functions and Memory

Coping and support in coping with the psychological distress and negative feelings such as anger, sadness, loneliness, confusion and fear[17] are the most frequently communicated self-reported needs of people with dementia living at home; they have been detected in more than half of studies.[6,7,9,17,27] Coping with memory problems is an area reported by people with dementia as one of the most commonly perceived unmet needs in two studies.[7,16]

2.3.6 Biological/Physical Needs: General Physical Health

General physical health includes requirements such as the need for dental care, specialist medical care, incontinence management and coping with polypharmacotherapy, eyesight and hearing problems compensation or support in solving malnutrition and dehydration problems.

Commutation of Chronic Health Problems. Poly-morbidity often results in polypharmacy, and a person with dementia often has no cognitive capacity to manage such a condition.[13] In the domain of pharmaceutical treatment and care,[11] the most reported need is treatment with anti-dementia drugs, which could also be a topic of discussion because of the limited effect of these drugs.[11] Unmet needs in general health and medical care were identified in three studies.[13,25,26] One study highlighted pharmaceutical treatment as an unmet need.[11] Eyesight/hearing problems management and compensation were specifically mentioned as an unmet need in three studies.[6,16,17,27] Sensory problems have a great influence on the ability to communicate (not only) for people with dementia. The unmet needs in eyesight/hearing indicate that a better treatment and/or compensation of these symptoms may enable better communication.[17]

2.3.7 Need for Safety

The care of home-dwelling people with dementia presents a great challenge, especially in ensuring safety. Safety issues may not be easily detected during formal care visits but may lead to a higher need for healthcare and a lower quality of life.[13] The need for safety,[25] specifically home and personal safety,[13] or environmental safety,[14] was reported as an important domain in three studies.[13,25,26] The most common need reported in this domain was avoiding the risk of falls,[13,25] wandering management,[25] and help with drug use.[13] Many people with dementia reported the need for a plan for dealing with emergencies (e.g., power outages)[13] or an emergency card for hospitalisation (which is a card identifying that the person has dementia and who their carers are and provides carer details).[11] The area of safety also includes safe driving, safe management of weapons and domestic tools[25] and prevention of abuse, neglect, or exploitation and fraud.[13] Accidental self-harm and creating dangerous situations unintentionally were listed as high in two studies.[6,27] Safety in the home and community and factors such as familiarity with surroundings, proximity of social support, safety and access to services were identified as reasons for wanting to remain living in their respective communities.[18]

2.4 Discussion

This scoping review provides a survey of self-reported needs of home-dwelling people with dementia. This population has been under-represented in research, even though meeting the individual needs of people with dementia is necessary for ensuring optimal care. The analysis of articles shows that people with dementia are able to express and communicate their needs themselves. Therefore, their experiences should be taken into account in person-centred care planning.

Needs and priorities in their perception are multi-dimensional and unique in each individual, and they change throughout life, vary according to the level of cognitive impairment and functional abilities and differ in the various subtypes and stages of dementia.[22,25] Needs assessment should include previous life experiences, cultural backgrounds, preferences and identity.[28] Therefore, when assessing self-reported needs, it is necessary to include the biological, psychological, social and environmental contexts of a person with dementia so that a unique assessment of that person's needs can be made to provide person-centred care.[22]

Environmental needs include a wide range of themes and specific topics in which people with dementia express their needs. The first theme is diagnosis and dementia evaluation. The onset of dementia syndrome is usually gradual and inconspicuous, and symptoms of the disease are often considered as regular aging. Initial symptoms of dementia are often unrecognised by people with dementia, their families and even health or social care professionals. Overlapping symptoms and poly-morbidity in older age make the diagnostic process even more difficult.[28] Another barrier to recognising dementia is that people with dementia often overestimate their abilities despite the actual state.[29] However, timely diagnosis is crucial for an appropriate assessment of the needs of a person with dementia and any changes that occur as the disease progresses.[30] Lack of communication between involved professionals and/or services occurs during the diagnostic process as well as during post-diagnostic support, which was another frequently occurring theme conveyed. Throughout the disease, access to information and coordination and continuity of care are identically identified as crucial. Furthermore, the access to non-pharmacological interventions and the need for dealing with legal issues and advance care planning were reported. An appropriate approach to meet these needs is case management.[28]

Other significant themes people with dementia reported include the need for company and meaningful roles and activities, as well as coping with psychological distress and the need for safety. Regardless of the need for division into themes, it can be assumed that if one main need is met, it will affect the perception of other needs. At some point, the fulfilled needs can drive away feelings of fear, sadness and anger and allow for a positive experience.[14] Because of communication difficulties, people with dementia may express their needs through non-normative behaviours. Evidence shows the link between behavioural and psychological symptoms in dementia (BPSD) and unmet needs,[31] for example, meaningful activities that focus on the individual interests and preserved skills of a person with dementia that increase that person's involvement, reduce BPSD and improve overall quality of life.[32] People with dementia express their needs through different behaviours, whereas a single type of behaviour can also convey different needs. The underlying needs associated with these behaviours thus must be understood before carrying out a person-centred care intervention.[32]

Biological needs are reported by people with dementia as a need for general and special medical care. One specific topic was the need for help with post-dementia changes, such as the ability to cope with drug management. The ageing of the population should be viewed as one of the main achievements of current healthcare. However, optimal management of healthcare for people with dementia is still a challenge that needs to be addressed in order to provide the basic human needs necessary to meet the full spectrum of individual needs and enable a person with dementia to live at home for as long as possible.

2.5 Implications

The findings presented in this scoping review provide an evidence-based framework that can serve as a guide in planning better care of people with dementia living at home. This review provides evidence that people with dementia are able to express their needs. Therefore, their perspective should be included in planning person-centred care together with a proxy account and observation.

2.6 Future Research

Several measurement tools have been used in quantitative studies to identify the needs of people with dementia; three of them were included in this scoping review (CANE, JHDCNA and the DelpHi Standard of Optimum Care). Each assessment described contained different domains and numbers of items, and comparing their results is almost impossible. This might be the reason for differences in numbers and frequency or even the existence of different needs reported in various studies. In addition, other findings and differences have been shown

in qualitative research. Further research on the needs of people with dementia, especially needs that those with dementia can formulate themselves, is still very necessary. An optimal needs-assessment instrument should assess needs comprehensively, be sensitive to change, allow re-evaluation of needs and leave additional space for written comments that go beyond the standardised needs items.[22]

2.7 Limitations

Four databases were used to search for articles; therefore, some articles may have been missed. The fact that most of the articles are in English can also mean that the results are more representative of a European or Western perspective.

2.8 Conclusion

The increasing numbers of people living with dementia need better support and care that can lead to a better quality of life. This review has shown that people with dementia themselves are important informants about their subjective needs and care experience, and therefore, they should not be neglected in research anymore. A total of five main themes were identified across the articles used in this scoping review. This provides evidence of a wide range of needs people with dementia experience in biological, psychological, social and environmental areas and the area of safety. To ensure optimal care, a comprehensive needs assessment in which the perceptions of people living with dementia are included is essential.

Disclosure Statement

The authors report no conflict of interest.

Funding

This study was supported by the Charles University Grant Agency, Project No. 760219.

References

1. World Health Organization (WHO). *Global Action Plan on the Public Health Response to Dementia 2017–2025*. Geneva: WHO; 2017.

2. Cohen-Mansfield J, Dakheel-Ali M, Marx MS, et al. Which unmet needs contribute to behavior problems in persons with advanced dementia? *Psychiatry Research* 2015; **228**(1):59–64.

3. Abreu W, Tolson D, Jackson GA, et al. The relationship between frailty, functional dependence, and healthcare needs among community-dwelling people with moderate to severe dementia. *Health & Social Care in the Community* 2019; **27**(3):642–53.

4. Schölzel-Dorenbos CJ, Meeuwsen EJ, Olde Rikkert MG. Integrating unmet needs into dementia health-related quality of life research and care: Introduction of the Hierarchy Model of Needs in Dementia. *Aging & Mental Health* 2010; **14**(1): 113–19.

5. van der Roest HG, Meiland FJ, Maroccini R, et al. Subjective needs of people with dementia: A review of the literature. *International Psychogeriatrics* 2007; **19**(3):559–92.

6. Miranda-Castillo C, Woods B, Galboda K, et al. Unmet needs, quality of life and support networks of people with dementia living at home. *Health and Quality of Life Outcomes* 2010; **8**(1):1–14.

7. van der Roest HG, Meiland FJ, Comijs HC, et al. What do community-dwelling people with dementia need? A survey of those who are known to care and welfare services. *International Psychogeriatrics* 2009; **21**(5):949–65.

8. Kerpershoek L, de Vugt M, Wolfs C, et al. Needs and quality of life of people with middle-stage dementia and their family carers from the European Actifcare study: When informal care alone may not suffice. *Aging & Mental Health* 2018; **22**(7):897–902.

9. Mazurek J, Szcześniak D, Urbańska K, et al. Met and unmet care needs of older people with dementia living at home: Personal and informal carers' perspectives. *Dementia* 2019; **18**(6):1963–75.

10. Scerri A, Scerri C, Innes A. The perceived and observed needs of patients with dementia admitted to acute medical wards. *Dementia* 2020; **19**(6): 1997–2017.

11. Eichler T, Thyrian JR, Hertel J, et al. Unmet needs of community-dwelling primary care patients with dementia in Germany: Prevalence and correlates. *Journal of Alzheimer's Disease* 2016; **51**(3):847–55.

12. Hansen A, Hauge S, Bergland Å. Meeting psychosocial needs for persons with dementia in home care services: A qualitative study of different perceptions and practices among health care providers. *BMC Geriatrics* 2017; **17**(1):1–10.

13. Black BS, Johnston D, Leoutsakos J, et al. Unmet needs in community-living persons with dementia are common, often non-medical and related to patient and caregiver characteristics. *International Psychogeriatrics* 2019; **31**(11):1643–54.

14. Kitwood T. The experience of dementia. *Aging & Mental Health* 1997; **1**(1):13–22.

15. Shiells K, Pivodic L, Holmerová I, van den Block L. Self-reported needs and experiences of people with dementia living in nursing homes: A scoping review. *Aging & Mental Health* 2019; **24** (10):1553–68.

16. Mazurek J, Szcześniak D, Lion KM, et al. Does the Meeting Centres Support Programme reduce unmet care needs of community-dwelling older people with dementia? A controlled, 6-month follow-up Polish study. *Clinical Interventions in Aging* 2019; 14:113–22.

17. Miranda-Castillo C, Woods B, Orrell M. The needs of people with dementia living at home from user, caregiver and professional perspectives: A cross-sectional survey. *BMC Health Services Research* 2013; **13**(1):1–10.

18. Morrisby C, Joosten A, Ciccarelli M. Needs of people with dementia and their spousal carers: A study of those living in the community. *Australasian Journal on Ageing* 2019; **38**(2):e43–9.

19. Colquhoun HL, Levac D, O'Brien KK, et al. Scoping reviews: Time for clarity in definition, methods, and reporting. *Journal of Clinical Epidemiology* 2014; **67**(12):1291–4.

20. Arksey H, O'Malley L. Scoping studies: Towards a methodological framework. *International Journal of Social Research Methodology* 2005; **8** (1):19–32.

21. Levac D, Colquhoun H, O'Brien KK. Scoping studies: Advancing the methodology. *Implementation Science* 2010; **5**(1):1–9.

22. Schmid R, Eschen A, Rüegger-Frey B, Martin M. Instruments for comprehensive needs assessment in individuals with cognitive complaints, mild cognitive impairment or dementia: A systematic review. *International Journal of Geriatric Psychiatry* 2012; **27**(4):329–41.

23. Disman, M. *Jak se vyrábí sociologická znalost: příručka pro uživatele*. Prague: Karolinum; 2000.

24. Górska S, Forsyth K, Irvine L, et al. Service-related needs of older people with dementia: Perspectives of service users and their unpaid carers. *International Psychogeriatrics* 2013; **25**(7):1107–14.

25. Black BS, Johnston D, Rabins PV, et al. Unmet needs of community-residing persons with dementia and their informal caregivers: Findings from the maximizing independence at home study. *Journal of the American Geriatrics Society* 2013; **61**(12):2087–95.

26. Johnston D, Samus QM, Morrison A, et al. Identification of community-residing individuals with dementia and their unmet needs for care.

International Journal of Geriatric Psychiatry 2011; **26**(3):292–8.

27. Miranda-Castillo C, Woods B, Orrell M. People with dementia living alone: What are their needs and what kind of support are they receiving? *International Psychogeriatrics* 2010; **22**(4):607–17.

28. Holmerová, I. *Case management v péči o lidi žijící s demencí: koordinace péče zaměřená na člověka*. Prague: Fakulta Humanitních Studií Univerzity Karlovy; 2018.

29. Machačová,K. Holmerová, I. *Aktivní gerontologie, aneb, Jak stárnout dobře*. Praha. Mladá fronta; 2019.

30. Iliffe S, Wilcock J, Synek M, et al. Case management for people with dementia and its translations: A discussion paper. *Dementia* 2019; **18**(3):951–69.

31. Algase DL, Beck C, Kolanowski A, et al. Need-driven dementia-compromised behavior: An alternative view of disruptive behavior. *American Journal of Alzheimer's Disease* 1996; **11**(6):10–19.

32. Sheppard CL, McArthur C, Hitzig SL. A systematic review of Montessori-based activities for persons with dementia. *Journal of the American Medical Directors Association* 2016; **17**(2):117–22.

Chapter 3

Needs of Older Primary Care Patients

Janine Stein and Steffi Gerlinde Riedel-Heller

3.1 Introduction

In old age, morbidity and the proportion of chronically ill patients in primary care increase. Because of multi-morbidity, older people belong to the population group with the highest use of medical services, and the general practitioner (GP) is usually the first contact point for older people.[1] According to current data, the age group between 70 and 79 years shows the highest levels of utilisation of primary care services (12-month prevalence) in registered doctors' practices with a population share of 83.4%.[2] Because GPs have the highest share of medical care, they play an important role in the care of somatic and mental illness in old age. In the field of mental health in old age, dementia and depression belong to the most common disorders. Further, cardiovascular diseases and musculoskeletal disorders are among the most common physical illnesses in individuals over 75 years of age.[3,4] These diseases cause not only great suffering for the affected patients but also high costs for the healthcare system. Older affected patients often have increased healthcare needs that may remain undetected and unmet. In order to ensure the best possible treatment and care for older patients, it is increasingly important that these needs are reliably detected and assessed. The assessment of patients' needs should involve multiple perspectives, including the perceptions of patients, family carers and healthcare professionals such as the GP. In this context, the Camberwell Assessment of Need for the Elderly (CANE) was developed to assess met and unmet needs. The CANE is particularly suitable for the multidimensional evaluation of medical and non-medical healthcare needs of older people from several perspectives.[5]

Since its development in 2004, the CANE has been used internationally in a variety of research contexts, samples and settings. In primary care, first investigations with the CANE were carried out in the United Kingdom by Walters et al.[6] A random sample of older GP patients aged 75 years and older, their relatives and medical staff were interviewed using the CANE. The most common unmet needs from the patients' perspective were eyesight/hearing/communication, psychological distress and continence. The three most common unmet needs from the relatives' point of view were mobility, eyesight/hearing/communication and accommodation. The most common unmet needs from the perspective of the medical staff were daytime activities, accommodation and mobility. Overall, the medical staff identified fewer unmet needs than patients and relatives. Thus, it can be assumed that there were unmet needs in this study that were not sufficiently recognised by the medical staff.[6] Another investigation using the CANE in older primary care patients was conducted in the Netherlands by Hoogendijk et al.[7] In this study, 1,137 frail older GP patients aged 65 years and older were interviewed with the CANE. The most common unmet needs were company (67.7%), daytime activities (48.4%), information (41.5%), caring for someone else (36.4%) and accommodation (34.3%). Regression analyses performed in this study showed that restrictions on the activities of daily living (ADLs) and increased frailty were strongly associated with unmet needs.[7] Further findings on met and unmet needs in primary care patients were reported by Stein et al.[8] In this study, the German version of the CANE was used to examine the needs of older GP patients from the perspectives of patients and their relatives. The most common met and unmet needs identified by patients and relatives were physical needs, including physical health, and eyesight/hearing/communication.[8]

Other studies in primary care using the CANE focused on common diseases in old age, such as dementia and depression. Miranda-Castillo et al.[9] interviewed older patients (60 years and older) with mild dementia living at home, their relatives and medical staff using the CANE. The most frequently reported unmet needs from the patients' perspective were psychological distress (21.6%), daytime activities (14.5%) and company (12.8%). There was a high agreement in terms of the kappa coefficient between the patients and the medical staff regarding met and unmet needs in the areas of deliberate self-harm ($\kappa = 0.83$) and intimate relationships ($\kappa = 0.77$). In nine CANE areas, good agreement was achieved with regard to met and unmet needs ($\kappa > 0.60$). A lower degree of agreement was observed in the CANE section for daytime activities ($\kappa = 0.21$). Good agreement between the patients and their relatives was evident in the CANE areas of eyesight/hearing/communication, mobility, continence, psychotic symptoms, deliberate self-harm and intimate relationships ($\kappa > 0.60$). With regard to all investigated CANE sections, the lowest agreement in met and unmet needs was found in daytime activities ($\kappa = 0.24$). Furthermore, Stein et al.[10] investigated the oldest old primary care patients (85+ years) with cognitive impairment and dementia, their relatives and GPs with regard to unmet needs. Most frequently, unmet needs were identified in the CANE sections for memory, looking after home and mobility. Risk factors for unmet needs in this patient group were a higher age, lower education and single marital status.[11] In addition, older primary care patients aged 75 years and older with and without depression were assessed using the CANE.[12] In this study, depressive older patients reported significantly more unmet needs than their healthy counterparts. Most frequently, needs in the sections for physical health, mobility/falls and company were reported as unmet by depressive patients. The levels of agreement between patients, relatives and GPs with regard to identified unmet needs varied between low and substantial and were higher in depressed patients and between patients and their relatives. It has been shown that the assessment of unmet needs of depressed older patients can vary widely across different assessment perspectives, which should be taken into account and brought into focus, especially in the primary care setting.[12] To date, it was not investigated what unmet needs older primary care patients with common somatic diseases such as cardiovascular diseases or musculoskeletal disorders report and how the needs appear compared to patients with the most common mental health disorders (dementia and depression).

3.2 Objectives of This Study

The aim of this study was to assess the needs of older primary care patients with the most common somatic and mental disorders. For this purpose, primary care patients aged 75 years and older ought to be interviewed using the adapted German version of the Camberwell Assessment of Need for the Elderly (CANE). In addition to the perspective of patients, their close relatives and their GPs should participate in the survey. The study should provide answers to the following research questions: What unmet needs do older primary care patients with cardiovascular diseases and musculoskeletal disorders (patients with primary diagnosis of somatic disorder) and with depression and dementia (patients with primary diagnosis of mental disorder) report? What unmet needs do their relatives and GPs report? What differences between the patient groups with regard to reported unmet needs can be observed?

3.3 Methods

3.3.1 Study Design

Data were collected in a study entitled, 'Needs Assessment in the Oldest Old: Application, Psychometric Examination and Establishment of the Adapted German Version of the Camberwell Assessment of Need for the Elderly (CANE)'. This study was funded by the German Research Foundation.

3.3.2 Procedure, Instruments and Sample

Patients were recruited via GP practices in Leipzig and the surrounding area. To participate in the study, the following criteria had to be fulfilled: (1) aged at least 75 years, (2) good or sufficient knowledge of German, (3) at least one GP visit within the last six months and (3) presence of at least one of the following primary diagnoses from the Tenth Revision of the *International Statistical Classification of Diseases and Related Health Problems* (ICD-10): cardiovascular diseases (I10–I15, I20–I25), musculoskeletal disorders (M15–M19, M40–M45, M80–M82), depression (F32–F33) and cognitive disorder or dementia (F00–F03, F05.1, G30–G31, R54). The following criteria led to exclusion from the study: (1) suicidality and (2) severe somatic diseases (e.g., final cancer stage). The GPs were asked to invite patients according to the given criteria for inclusion and exclusion as well to inform them about the study. Eligible patients completed a written informed consent. Subsequently, the patients were contacted by the study staff of the University of Leipzig to make an appointment for the personal interview. Patients were interviewed using a structured interview that included the adapted German version of the CANE.[13] In addition, socio-demographic information on age, gender, marital status, education, vocational training and domicile was collected. The standardised interviews were conducted by trained psychologists and health scientists in the home surroundings of the patients and on request also in the study centre or in the GP practices. If eligible, the relatives of the patients were invited to participate in the study. After a brief consultation with the study staff, they were also asked to sign a written informed consent form. The structured interviews of relatives were conducted either personally, by telephone or in writing. Additionally, the participating GPs were interviewed in writing with regard to the needs of their patients by means of a questionnaire containing the CANE.

In total, 100 psychiatric patients (n = 50 patients with dementia, n = 50 patients with depression) and 100 somatic patients with cardiovascular diseases (n = 50 patients with either hypertension, angina pectoris, myocardial infarction, or chronic ischemic heart disease) as well as with musculoskeletal disorders (n = 50 patients with osteoarthritis or osteoporosis) were recruited and asked about their needs.

3.3.3 Statistical Analyses

Patients were assigned to one of the following groups according to their primary ICD-10 diagnosis: cardiovascular disease, musculoskeletal disease, depression and dementia. Patients with multi-morbidity were classified as dementia patients in the presence of dementia, although other diagnoses such as cardiovascular diseases coexisted. Similarly, patients with depression and co-morbid illnesses other than dementia have been included in the group of depressive patients. Patients who had both cardiovascular and musculoskeletal disorders were classified into either musculoskeletal disorders (n = 38) or cardiovascular diseases (n = 11), so the sample sizes of somatic patients were equal.

To examine the distribution of met and unmet needs from the perspectives of patients, relatives and GPs, descriptive analyses in terms of mean ± standard deviations or frequencies with percentages were performed. For this purpose, a sum score for unmet needs was created for each CANE section and for the CANE categories physical, psychological, environmental and social needs. Analyses were run for the total sample and for the disease-specific subgroups. In order to determine differences between the various disease groups in terms of socio-demographic data, chi-squared tests were carried out or with a cell size of $n \le 5$ Fisher's exact tests for qualitative variables and Kruskal–Wallis tests for quantitative variables (age). The socio-demographic data were age, gender, marital status (single/divorced, married, widowed), school education (no school-leaving certificate or general elementary education, intermediate school-leaving certificate, polytechnic secondary school-leaving certificate), vocational education (no vocational education, apprenticeship, vocational school certificate, technical college/university degree) and domicile (alone, living together with spouse/partner, living together with others, assisted living/nursing home).

3.3.4 Results

For the survey, a total of 260 patients could be recruited via participating GP practices. Of these, 29 patients were excluded from the investigation because they either withdrew their participation (n = 20), were no longer attainable (n = 6), did not meet the age criterion of at least 75 years (n = 1), could not be interviewed because of significant cognitive impairment (n = 1) or were deceased (n = 1). The analysis sample consisted of 231 patients. GP information was available for all patients (n = 231), and 168 interviews with close relatives could be conducted. The sub-samples consisted of 51 patients with cardiovascular diseases (22.08%) and 51 patients with musculoskeletal disorders (22.08%). Further, 65 patients with depression (28.14%) and 64 patients with dementia (27.70%) were interviewed.

Table 3.1 shows the socio-demographic data of the patients. The average age was 81.85 years (standard deviation [SD] = 5.03). About two-thirds (n = 155, 67.10%) of the total sample were female. About 45.45% (n = 105) were widowed, 42.42% (n = 98) were married and 12.12% (n = 28) were single or divorced. Half the patients (n = 115, 49.78%) had an intermediate school-leaving certificate, a quarter of the patients had no school-leaving certificate or general elementary education (n = 59, 25.54%) and another quarter had an advanced technical college certificate or the Abitur (n = 57, 24.68%). More than a third of the patients had completed an apprenticeship (n = 83, 35.93%), 28.14% (n = 65) had completed the vocational school degree and 25.11% (n = 58) had a college or university degree. Most patients lived

Table 3.1 Socio-demographic Characteristics of Patients

Characteristic	Total	CVD	MSD	Depression	Dementia	χ^2	p-Value
Sample size, n (%)	231 (100)	51 (22.08)	51 (22.08)	65 (28.14)	64 (27.71)		
Age, yrs (M, SD)	81.85 (5.03)	81.27 (5.30)	81.39 (4.68)	81.02 (4.25)	83.53 (5.52)	8.86	0.031
Gender, n (%)							
Male	76 (32.90)	20 (39.22)	18 (35.29)	16 (24.62)	22 (34.38)	3.14	0.371
Female	155 (67.10)	31 (60.78)	33 (64.71)	49 (75.38)	42 (65.63)	3.14	0.371
Marital status, n (%)							
Single/divorced	28 (12.12)	4 (7.84)	5 (9.80)	7 (10.77)	12 (18.75)	FE	0.324
Married	98 (42.42)	24 (47.06)	21 (41.18)	26 (40.00)	27 (42.19)	0.64	0.887
Widowed	105 (45.45)	23 (45.10)	25 (49.02)	32 (49.23)	25 (39.06)	1.69	0.639
School education, n (%)							
No school-leaving certificate/general elementary education	59 (25.54)	13 (25.49)	13 (25.49)	14 (21.54)	19 (29.69)	1.13	0.771
Intermediate school-leaving certificate/polytechnic secondary school	115 (49.78)	21 (41.18)	23 (45.10)	40 (61.54)	31 (48.44)	5.60	0.133
Advanced technical college certificate/Abitur	57 (24.68)	17 (33.33)	15 (29.41)	11 (16.92)	14 (21.88)	5.04	0.169
Vocational education, n (%)							
No vocational education	25 (10.82)	1 (1.96)	4 (7.84)	5 (7.69)	15 (23.44)	FE	0.002
Apprenticeship	83 (35.93)	18 (35.29)	13 (25.49)	30 (46.15)	22 (34.38)	5.44	0.142
Vocational school certificate	65 (28.14)	14 (27.45)	18 (35.29)	20 (30.77)	13 (20.31)	3.46	0.325
Technical college/university degree	58 (25.11)	18 (35.29)	16 (31.37)	10 (15.38)	14 (21.88)	7.50	0.057
Domicile, n (%)							
Alone	101 (43.72)	22 (43.14)	27 (52.94)	28 (43.08)	24 (37.50)	2.79	0.426
With spouse/partner	99 (42.86)	25 (49.02)	22 (43.14)	27 (41.54)	25 (39.06)	1.22	0.749
With others	10 (4.33)	1 (1.96)	1 (1.96)	1 (1.54)	7 (10.94)	FE	0.047
Assisted living/nursing home	21 (9.09)	3 (5.88)	1 (1.96)	9 (13.85)	8 (12.50)	FE	0.073

Notes: Total = total sample of patients; CVD = subsample of patients with cardiovascular diseases; MSD = subsample of patients with musculoskeletal disorders; Depression = subsample of patients with depression; Dementia = subsample of patients with cognitive impairment or dementia; χ^2 = chi-squared test, Pearson chi-squared tests (qualitative variables) or Kruskal–Wallis test (age) for the evaluation of subsample differences; p-value = level of significance (if cell size ≤ 5 corrected with FE = Fisher's exact test); n = sample size; M = mean; SD = standard deviation.

either alone (n = 101, 43.72%) or with their partner (n = 99, 42.86%). Subgroup analyses revealed significant differences regarding age, vocational training and living situation. In particular, it was found that the group of patients with dementia was, on average, about two years older than those of the other subgroups, lived more often with others and were more frequently without a degree.

3.4 Unmet Needs from the Patients' Perspective

Overall, the most frequent needs (total needs) were reported in the areas of eyesight/hearing/communication (n = 212, 92.58%), physical health (n = 185, 80.79%), mobility (n = 132, 57, 64%), mobility/falls (n = 92, 40.18%) and continence (n = 90, 39.30%). With regard to unmet needs, the most needs that were reported were in the physical need's category (n = 128, 41.97%), followed by unmet social (n = 67, 21.97%), environmental (n = 57, 18.69%) and psychological (n = 53, 17.38%) needs. Figure 3.1 illustrates the frequency of unmet needs from the patients' perspective in each CANE section. Most frequently, unmet needs were reported in the CANE sections for physical health (n = 36, 15.72%), information (n = 26, 11.40%), mobility (n = 26, 11.35%), eyesight/hearing/communication (n = 22, 9.61%) and accommodation (n = 22, 9.61%).

No unmet needs were reported with regard to psychotic symptoms. In addition, only one unmet need (n = 1, 0.44%) was expressed in the section for caring for someone else, alcohol, and abuse/neglect.

Figure 3.2 shows the 10 most commonly reported unmet needs from the patients' perspective across the four disease-specific subgroups. Overall, the most common unmet needs were reported in the area of physical health, followed by information and mobility. Patients with somatic diseases reported fewer unmet needs than patients with mental illness. Particularly in the subgroup with cardiovascular diseases, the proportion of patients with unmet needs was comparatively low. For example, only 2 patients with cardiovascular diseases (4%) reported physical needs as being unmet, whereas 15 patients with depression (23%) reported unmet physical needs.

In all subgroups, physical needs accounted for the largest share of unmet needs (35%–57%). Eleven unmet physical needs (44%) were reported in patients with cardiovascular disease, 31 in patients with musculoskeletal disorders (57%), 48 in the subgroup of patients with depression (41%) and 38 in dementia patients (35%). In addition, in the subgroups of depression and dementia patients, 26 (22%) and 20 (18%) unmet psychological needs were expressed, whereas in the subgroups of cardiovascular and musculoskeletal disease patients,

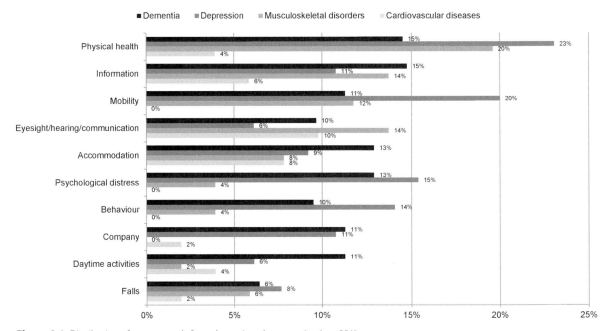

Figure 3.1 Distribution of unmet needs from the patients' perspective (n = 231)

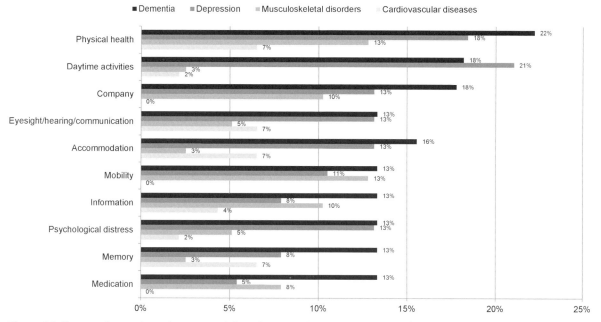

Figure 3.2 Ten most frequently rated unmet needs from the patients' perspective across the four disease-specific subgroups

only 1 (4%) and 6 (11%) unmet psychological needs were reported. Patients with mental illness also reported significantly more unmet needs in the categories of environmental ($n = 43$ versus $n = 14$) and social needs ($n = 51$ versus $n = 16$) than patients with somatic diseases.

3.5 Unmet Needs from the Relatives' Perspective

Similar to the patient survey, most needs (total needs) of patients were identified by their relatives in the sections for eyesight/hearing/communication ($n = 145$, 86.31%), physical health ($n = 143$, 85.12%) and mobility ($n = 91$, 54.17%). Correspondingly, relatives also reported the most unmet needs in the category of physical needs ($n = 89$, 38.36%), followed by social ($n = 58$, 25.00%), environmental ($n = 44$, 18.97%) and psychological needs ($n = 41$, 17.67%). Most of the unmet needs were reported in the CANE sections for physical health ($n = 25$, 14.88%), daytime activities ($n = 18$, 10.78%), company ($n = 17$, 10.12%) and eyesight/hearing/communication and accommodation (in each case $n = 16$, 9.52%). In addition, only one unmet need ($n = 1$, 0.60%) was expressed in the areas of money/budgeting and alcohol. No unmet needs were identified in the areas of deliberate self-harm and abuse/neglect.

Figure 3.3 shows the 10 most common unmet needs of patients from the perspective of their relatives across the four disease-specific subgroups. Most frequently, unmet needs were detected in the area of physical health, followed by daytime activities and company. Along with the patients' perspective, relatives expressed fewer unmet needs for patients with somatic diseases than for those with mental illness. Particularly in the subgroup of cardiovascular diseases, the proportion of unmet needs was comparatively lower. For example, for only 2% ($n = 1$) of patients with cardiovascular disease did the relatives report unmet needs in the CANE section involving daytime activities, whereas for patients with depression, this share was 21% ($n = 8$).

3.6 Unmet Needs from the GPs' Perspective

Overall, fewer unmet needs were identified by GPs than by patients and relatives. Most needs (total needs) were identified in the areas of physical health ($n = 190$, 83.34%), psychological distress ($n = 119$, 51.52%), looking after home ($n = 101$, 43.72%), eyesight/hearing/communication ($n = 99$, 42.86%) and continence ($n = 89$, 38.53%). In contrast to the ratings of patients and relatives, GPs most frequently reported unmet needs in terms of psychological needs ($n = 51$, 31.68%), followed

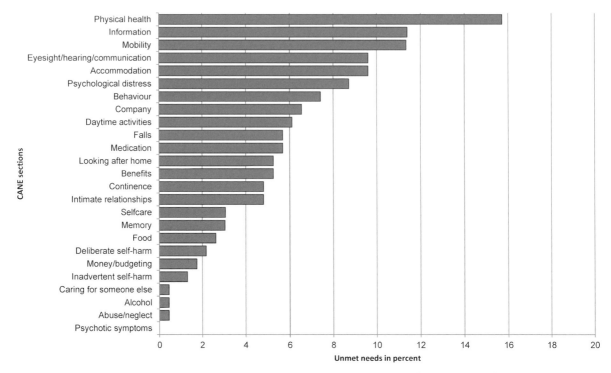

Figure 3.3 Ten most frequently rated unmet needs from the relatives' perspective across the four disease-specific subgroups

by social (n = 44, 27.33%), physical (n = 39, 24.22%) and environmental needs (n = 27, 16.77%). Most of the patients' unmet needs were reported by GPs in the areas of psychological distress (n = 21, 9.09%), company (n = 18, 7.86%), daytime activities (n = 15, 6.58%), physical health (n = 10, 4.39%) and behaviour (n = 10, 4.37%).

Figure 3.4 shows the 10 most common unmet needs of patients from the GPs' point of view for the four disease-specific subgroups. Needs in the area of psychological distress were most frequently rated as unmet by GPs, followed by company and daytime activities. From the perspective of GPs, patients with somatic diseases also showed fewer unmet needs than patients with mental illness. In the section for psychological distress, for example, GPs reported that only 4% (n = 2) of patients with cardiovascular disease had unmet needs, whereas for those with depression, the amount of perceived unmet needs was 14% (n = 9).

Overall, GPs identified significantly fewer unmet needs than relatives and patients themselves. For example, in the group of patients with cardiovascular diseases, about 10% of patients (n = 5 of 51) and 7% of relatives (n = 3 of 46) reported unmet needs in the

CANE section for eyesight/hearing/communication, whereas none of the GPs identified reported unmet needs in this area. The patients' and relatives' perceptions of needs were very similar for all disease groups, with some exceptions. For example, only about 6% (n = 4 of 65) of patients with depression reported unmet needs in the section for daytime activities, whereas 21% (n = 8 of 38) of their relatives identified unmet needs. In addition, in the group of patients with cardiovascular diseases, fewer unmet needs were reported than in the other disease groups. The needs situations of patients with dementia and depression differed only marginally.

3.7 Discussion

The aim of this study was to analyse the unmet needs of older primary care patients with the most common somatic and mental illnesses. For this purpose, the patients' own perspective was recorded, as well as the perspectives of their relatives and GPs, using the adapted German version of the Camberwell Assessment of Need for the Elderly (CANE). The results show that most of the unmet needs were reported from the perspectives of patients and

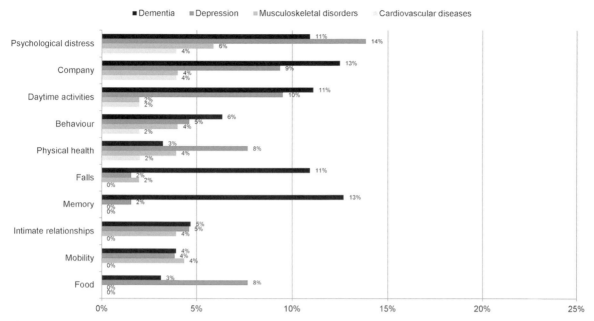

Figure 3.4 Ten most frequently rated unmet needs from the GPs´ perspective across the four disease-specific subgroups

relatives in the category of physical needs regardless of whether the patients' primary medical diagnosis was a somatic or mental disorder. Thus, the most common unmet need from the patients' and relatives' perspectives was reported in the area of physical health. In addition, from the patients´ point of view, the sections for information and mobility were among the most common unmet needs, whereas relatives identified the needs in the sections for daytime activities and company as unmet. Overall, patients with mental illness expressed more unmet needs than patients with somatic disorders, especially patients with cardiovascular disease. GPs reported the most common unmet needs in the category of psychological needs, such as psychological distress, behaviour and memory.

3.8 Frequencies and Distribution of Needs in Old Age from the Perspective of Patients, Relatives and GPs

Consistent with a study that also used the CANE in a sample of 1,137 older primary care patients with an average age of 81 years, physical health, mobility and eyesight/hearing/communication were among the most common overall patient needs.[7] In addition,

the area of looking after home was one of the five most common needs in the study by Hoogendijk et al.[7] However, only 13 CANE sections were assessed in their study, which limits the comparability with the results reported here. In this study, continence was one of the five most frequently reported needs, which was also reported as one of the most common needs in the general older population aged 75 years and above.[14]

The most frequently identified unmet needs of patients in this study are at least partially comparable with previous findings in primary care. For example, in a previous study using the CANE in older primary care patients (65+ years), physical health, mobility and eyesight/hearing/communication were among the most commonly observed unmet needs.[15] Moreover, Smith and Orrell[15] found the patients' psychological distress among the most common unmet needs, which was also demonstrated in another study of GP patients aged 75 years and older interviewed with the CANE.[6] Although psychological distress has been identified by GPs as the most common unmet need in this study, it was not identified as one of the most common unmet needs from the perspectives of patients or relatives. The GPs in this study also identified company and daytime activities as the most common unmet needs of patients, which were also ranked among the top five unmet needs from the perspective of the medical staff in the study by Walters et al.[6] By contrast, needs in accommodation and mobility were compared to the study of Walters et al.[6] and were rarely identified as unmet by GPs. Further discrepancies between this study and that by Walters et al.[6] with regard to the perspective of relatives were observed. Whereas the latter mainly found unmet needs for mobility, eyesight/hearing/communication and accommodation from the relatives' point of view, the relatives in this study reported unmet needs particularly in the patients' physical health, daytime activities and company. Walters et al.[6] pointed out that healthcare professionals recognised relatively few of the unmet needs identified by patients themselves. As a possible explanation, they argued that healthcare professionals may have a different understanding of the concept of need or have divergent information about patients' lives. This would also explain why the views of patients and relatives in this study were closer to each other in terms of perceived unmet needs than those of patients and GPs.

3.9 Subgroup Differences Regarding Unmet Needs

In all four subgroups, the areas of physical health and information were among the most frequently stated unmet needs from the patients' perspective. Mobility was one of the five most common unmet needs in all subgroups, with the exception of the subgroup of patients with cardiovascular diseases. In addition, the CANE section looking after home appeared to be one of the five most commonly mentioned unmet needs in the subgroups of patients with cardiovascular diseases, musculoskeletal disorders and dementia. In the samples with a primary somatic diagnosis, the area of eyesight/hearing/communication was one of the five most common unmet needs compared to patients with a primary mental health diagnosis. Patients with dementia or depression, by contrast, were more likely to report unmet needs in the areas of psychological distress and behaviour than patients with a somatic disorder. Overall, the subgroups of patients with mental illness reported significantly more unmet needs than patients with impaired physical health. Whereas patients with cardiovascular diseases reported the fewest unmet needs, the most unmet

needs were observed in the subgroup of patients with depression. In the following, we will discuss similarities and differences between the subgroups, taking into account past research findings.

So far, care needs of older people in samples of older patients with primary somatic diagnoses were rarely explored. Thus, for the first time, this study describes the need situation of older primary care patients with cardiovascular and musculoskeletal disorders as assessed using the CANE. A previous study investigated the needs of patients with suspected myocardial infarction using the Nottingham Health Needs Assessment (NHNA) tool. However, the NHNA differs greatly from the CANE in that it largely ignores psychological needs and mainly addresses physical, informational and social needs. In the NHNA study, problems in social areas were most frequently reported in a sample of 242 patients at the average age of 70 years. The authors emphasised that social factors such as living alone and social isolation require special attention in the care of older cardiac patients.[16]

Overall, patients with somatic disorders, especially with cardiovascular diseases, showed significantly fewer unmet needs than patients from the other subgroups in this study. One explanation could be that the group of patients with cardiovascular diseases also included patients with hypertension. Although hypertension is related to severe health consequences, it can remain unnoticed for a long time and therefore does not necessarily cause any impairments, which could be related to fewer perceived unmet needs.[17] By contrast, it may be easier to identify and address the needs of patients with somatic versus mental diseases. Consequently, those patients can be better provided with healthcare. Earlier studies argued that mental illnesses such as depression are often not recognised in old age, not least because of co-morbidities and occurring somatic symptoms.[18,19] Thus, it may be more difficult to detect and address the needs of patients with mental disorders compared to patients with somatic disorders. Past studies showed that even patients with diagnosed depression often remain untreated.[20] Although older patients with depression often benefit from healthcare services, only a small proportion of those affected receive depression-specific treatment.[21] This could lead to unmet needs in many different areas in this patient group. In the past, needs assessment was more frequently conducted in older samples with mental disorders such as depression[11,22–24] or cognitive impairment and dementia.[9,10,25,26] For example, Stein et al.[11] reported in a multicenter study in the German primary care setting that older patients with depression mainly reported unmet needs in the areas of physical health, mobility, company, psychological distress and daytime activities, which is largely in line with the results reported here. According to the authors, the high occurrence of unmet physical needs could be due to the facts that depression is often masked by physical symptoms and that depressive syndromes occur more frequently in patients with physical complaints such as chronic pain.[27] In comparison, needs in the area of psychological distress were identified most commonly as unmet in a psychiatric sample of older adults with depression.[23] These results may be attributed to different sample characteristics and diagnostic approaches. Whereas participants in the study by Houtjes et al.[23] were diagnosed with a major depression by a psychiatrist and treated on an outpatient basis, this study was based on GP diagnoses and included patients with milder forms of depressive disorders. Furthermore, previous studies reported that subjects with depression or depressive symptoms reported significantly more unmet needs than those without depression.[24,28] Along with this, many studies found that depression in old age is associated with reduced quality of life[29] and other negative consequences, such as social isolation; limited physical, cognitive and social functioning; and increased suicidality and morbidity.[30–32] As a serious burden in old age, depression is likely to negatively affect the needs of older patients. By contrast, needs that are not identified and addressed could also cause depressive symptoms. For example, in a longitudinal study of 4,162 older adults, the perception of basic unmet needs predicted depressive symptoms over a 10-year span. Therefore, unmet needs should be addressed early to prevent a possible onset of depressive symptoms and disorders.[33] In this context, the GPs play an important role in often being the first point of contact for older people suffering from depression.

According to previous studies and in line with the current findings, patients with dementia have also reported more unmet needs than unaffected patients.[34,35] Likewise, our data show that patients with dementia have more unmet needs than patients with somatic diseases. Partly in line with our findings, previous studies with dementia patients also identified the most common unmet needs in the categories of social needs such as information,[25,36] physical needs such as mobility[10] and psychological needs such as memory or psychological distress,[9,10,25,34,37,38] even if the studies can only be compared to a limited extent. In a recent study, relatives and GPs of patients with dementia reported more unmet needs than the patients themselves.[10] This finding has also been confirmed in previous studies.[9,34] In other studies, the number of reported unmet needs was similar regardless of the perspective of the patients or healthcare professionals.[36,37] However, the comparability of results is limited because of different samples and settings. In primary care, this discrepancy is most notable in the study by Stein et al.[10] In their study, older patients with mild cognitive impairment did not report any unmet needs, whereas their relatives and GPs identified numerous unmet needs for this patient group. In line with these findings, patients with dementia reported fewer unmet needs in the memory section compared to their relatives and GPs in this study. This could be due to a lack of insight, denial or a lack of awareness of the patients' own memory problems, a phenomenon known as anosognosia.[39] However, there are conflicting findings with regard to anosognosia in patients with cognitive impairment,[40] and the reasons that may cause the observed discrepancies between patients´ and GPs´ perceptions of unmet needs remain unclear. Consequently, information on needs from the point of view of patients with cognitive impairment should generally be interpreted with caution. Nevertheless, an early needs assessment in patients with incipient dementia from different perspectives would be desirable. Thus, tailored treatment could be initiated at an early stage, which may have a positive effect on the course of the disease. Further, in this study, unmet needs in the CANE section for information were identified as most common in patients with dementia and were also among the most common unmet needs in all other subgroups. As has been suggested in the past, the provision of disease-related information and treatment options for older patients with cognitive impairment and dementia in primary care should be improved.[15,41] This can be a first important step to address the unmet needs of patients with dementia and other common diseases of old age. Improved patient education may also have a positive impact on other areas where unmet needs exist.

One strength of this study is that in contrast to many previous studies, it included patients with a mental illness as well as patients with primary somatic diseases. Thus, this study allowed a direct comparison of the needs of subgroups with depressive disorders, dementia, musculoskeletal disorders and cardiovascular diseases. In addition, a sample of patients aged 75 years and older was examined. This age group represents an increasing proportion of the population and should be given special attention with regard to unmet care needs. Another strength of this study is the assessment of needs from different perspectives, including the patients themselves, their relatives and GPs. This procedure provided complementary information and may have prevented possible distortions by socially desirable patient responses. Subgroup-specific tendencies were derived that are relevant for early addressing of unmet needs and the initiation of targeted interventions. Whereas multi-morbidity is a widespread condition in old age,[42] the investigated samples are representative of older populations with common diseases.

3.10 Conclusion and Future Directions

Overall, it has been shown that older groups of patients with the most common somatic and mental diseases have specific unmet needs. These should be considered in primary, clinical and nursing care of older patients. Suitable instruments such as the CANE should be used to reliably and validly assess the needs. On this basis, implications for the health and social care of older patients should be derived, appropriate treatment should be initiated or relevant information should be made available. A valid needs assessment may be the basis for targeted interventions and thus represents an important starting point for the healthcare of older people. The results of this study may substantially improve the care situation of older GP patients with common somatic and mental diseases.

However, needs assessment in older primary care patients can be challenging in terms of using a tool that is appropriate for older people and also suitable for use in routine consultations in general practice. Based on the original version of the CANE, initial efforts were made in the United Kingdom to develop a short instrument for the fast and economical assessment of particularly relevant care needs in primary care. The results show that certain areas of need (e.g., eyesight/hearing, physical health, mobility, continence, cognition and psychological distress)

have been most frequently identified as being unmet in older primary care patients. Based on these findings, a shorter version with five priority domains was developed (SPICE): Senses, Physical ability, Incontinence, Cognition and Emotional distress.[43] Most recently, the SPICE tool was evaluated by Balsinha et al.[44] (2018) in a mixed-methods study in Portugal taking into account the perspectives of both GPs and patients. In this study, the SPICE interview was completed by older patients and their GPs. Further, perceptions about its use in primary care were explored. The authors found that emotional distress was the most frequent unmet need reported by patients. The study showed that the SPICE tool yielded valuable information and significantly helped to identify unmet needs of older people in primary care. Overall, it was well accepted by both patients and GPs. However, the practical application of SPICE should be further evaluated, and its implementation may require facilitating strategies.[44]

In the future, studies should further examine the needs of these patient groups from different perspectives in larger-scale longitudinal studies and identify factors that influence the occurrence of unmet needs. A longitudinal study would make it possible to better understand the relationship between risk factors and unmet needs. In future studies, however, not only risk factors for unmet needs but also protective factors should be brought into focus. In addition, it should be examined to what extent the early addressing of unmet needs affects the course of the disease and the quality of life of patients. From the patients' point of view, the most frequently reported unmet needs were in the areas of physical health, information and mobility. How can addressing these unmet needs improve the health of patients with depression or slow down the progression of dementia? This question requires further evaluation and consideration. Especially in the area of information, the provision of information brochures or targeted interventions for an improved doctor-patient communication may address many unmet needs of patients. In addition, the needs of those affected should be assessed from different perspectives. In this way, a holistic care concept can be developed for the individual patient, taking into account relevant needs from the point of view of patients themselves, relatives and healthcare professionals. In this context, it should be remembered that data collection from several perspectives is challenging because patients may sometimes give socially desirable responses or, in the case of cognitive disorders, have a lack of insight into the disease and their unmet needs. In addition, the results of this study represent a starting point for further research. In particular, gender differences and the role of partnership status or widowhood should be further explored in this context. Last but not least, the expectations that patients have towards the healthcare system may also depend on whether they perceive their needs as met or unmet.

Acknowledgements

This study was funded by the German Research Foundation under Grant No. STE 2235/1–2 and under Grant No. RI 1856/4–2. Janine Stein was supported by the German Federal Ministry of Education and Research under Grant No. 01GY1613. We want to thank all participants for their good collaboration.

References

1. Glaesmer H, Gunzelmann T, Martin A, et al. The impact of mental disorders on health care utilization and illness behaviour in the elderly. *Psychiatric Praxis* 2008; **35**(4):187–93.

2. Rattay P, Butschalowsky H, Rommel A, et al. Utilization of outpatient and inpatient health services in Germany: Results of the German Health Interview and Examination Survey for Adults (DEGS1). *Bundesgesundheitsblatt Gesundheitsforschung Gesundheitsschutz* 2013; **56**(5–6):832–44.

3. Fuchs J, Busch M, Lange C, Scheidt-Nave C. Prevalence and patterns of morbidity among adults in Germany: Results of the German telephone health interview survey German Health Update (GEDA) 2009. *Bundesgesundheitsblatt Gesundheitsforschung Gesundheitsschutz* 2012; **55**(4):576–86.

4. Fuchs J, Rabenberg M, Scheidt-Nave C. Prevalence of selected musculoskeletal conditions in Germany: Results of the German Health Interview and Examination Survey for Adults (DEGS1). *Bundesgesundheitsblatt Gesundheitsforschung Gesundheitsschutz* 2013; **56**(5–6):678–86.

5. Orrell M, Hancock G. *CANE: Camberwell Assessment of Need for the Elderly*. New York: Gaskell; 2004.

6. Walters K, Iliffe S, Tai SS, Orrell M. Assessing needs from patient, carer and professional perspectives: The Camberwell Assessment of Need for Elderly people in primary care. *Age Ageing* 2000; **29**(6):505–10.

7. Hoogendijk EO, Muntinga ME, van Leeuwen KM, et al. Self-perceived met and unmet care needs of frail older adults in primary care. *Archives of Gerontology and Geriatrics* 2014; **58**(1):37–42.

8. Stein J, Luppa M, König H-H, Riedel-Heller SG. Assessing met and unmet needs in the oldest-old and psychometric properties of the German version of the Camberwell Assessment of Need for the Elderly (CANE): A pilot study. *International Psychogeriatrics* 2014; **26**(2):285–95.

9. Miranda-Castillo C, Woods B, Orrell M. The needs of people with dementia living at home from user, caregiver and professional perspectives: A cross-sectional survey. *BMC Health Services Research* 2013; **13**:1–10.

10. Stein J, Pabst A, Luck T, et al. Unmet care needs in the oldest old primary care patients with cognitive disorders: Results of the AgeCoDe and AgeQualiDe study. *Dementia and Geriatric Cognitive Disorders* 2017; **44**(1–2):71–83.

11. Stein J, Pabst A, Weyerer S, et al. The assessment of met and unmet care needs in the oldest old with and without depression using the Camberwell Assessment of Need for the Elderly (CANE): Results of the AgeMooDe study. *Journal of Affective Disorders* 2016; **193**:309–17.

12. Stein J, Pabst A, Weyerer S, et al. Unmet care needs of the oldest old with late-life depression: A comparison of patient, caring relative and general practitioner perceptions—Results of the AgeMooDe study. *Journal of Affective Disorders* 2016; **205**:182–9.

13. Stein J, Dorow M, Liegert P, et al. *Camberwell Assessment of Need for the Elderly (CANE): Handbuch für die adaptierte deutsche Version*, 1st ed. Cologne: Psychiatrie Verlag; 2019.

14. Stein J, Liegert P, Dorow M, et al. Unmet health care needs in old age and their association with depression: Results of a population-representative survey. *Journal of Affective Disorders* 2019; **245**: 998–1006.

15. Smith F, Orrell M. Does the patient-centred approach help identify the needs of older people attending primary care? *Age & Ageing* 2007; **36**(6):628–31.

16. Asadi-Lari M, Packham C, Gray D. Unmet health needs in patients with coronary heart disease: Implications and potential for improvement in caring services. *Health and Quality of Life Outcomes* 2003; **1**:1–8.

17. Raji YR, Abiona T, Gureje O. Awareness of hypertension and its impact on blood pressure control among elderly Nigerians: Report from the Ibadan study of aging. *Pan African Medical Journal* 2017; **27**:1–14.

18. Mitchell AJ, Rao S, Vaze A. Do primary care physicians have particular difficulty identifying late-life depression? A meta-analysis stratified by age. *Psychotherapy and Psychosomatics* 2010; **79**(5): 285–94.

19. Kok RM, Reynolds CF. Management of depression in older adults: A review. *Journal of the American Medical Association* 2017; **317**(20):2114–22.

20. Wittchen H-U, Jacobi F. Met and unmet needs for intervention: Clinical-epidemiological estimations for mental disorders in the German Health Interview and Examination Survey Supplement. *Bundesgesundheitsblatt Gesundheitsforschung Gesundheitsschutz* 2001; **44**(10):993–1000.

21. Busch MA, Neuner B, Aichberger MC, et al. Depressive symptomatik und inanspruchnahme von gesundheits- und pflegeleistungen bei personen im alter ab 50 Jahren in Deutschland: Ergebnisse einer bevölkerungsbasierten Querschnittstudie. *Psychiatric Praxis* 2013; **40**(4):214–19.

22. Hancock GA, Reynolds T, Woods B, et al. The needs of older people with mental health problems according to the user, the carer, and the staff. *International Journal of Geriatric Psychiatry* 2003; **18**(9):803–11.

23. Houtjes W, van Meijel B, Deeg DJH, Beekman ATF. Major depressive disorder in late life: A multifocus perspective on care needs. *Aging & Mental Health* 2010; **14**(7):874–80.

24. Alltag S, Stein J, Pabst A, et al. Unmet needs in the depressed primary care elderly and their relation to severity of depression: Results from the AgeMooDe study. *Aging & Mental Health* 2017; **22**(8):1032–9.

25. van der Roest HG, Meiland FJM, Comijs HC, et al. What do community-dwelling people with dementia need? A survey of those who are known to care and welfare services. *International Psychogeriatrics* 2009; **21**(5):949–65.

26. Passos J, Sequeira C, Fernandes L. The needs of older people with mental health problems: A particular focus on dementia patients and their carers. *International Journal of Alzheimers Disease* 2012; 2012:1–7.

27. Zainab AM, Pereira XV. Depression in primary care: Part 1. Screening and diagnosis. *Malaysian Family Physician: The Official Journal of the Academy of Family Physicians of Malaysia* 2007; **2**(3):95–101.

28. Futeran S, Draper BM. An examination of the needs of older patients with chronic mental illness in public mental health services. *Aginging & Mental Health* 2012; **16**(3):327–34.

29. Sivertsen H, Bjørkløf GH, Engedal K, et al. Depression and quality of life in older persons: A review. *Dementia and Geriatric Cognitive Disorders* 2015; **40**(5–6):311–39.

30. Hybels CF, Blazer DG, Pieper CF. Toward a threshold for subthreshold depression: An analysis of correlates of depression by severity of symptoms using data from an elderly community sample. *Gerontologist* 2001; **41**(3):357–65.

31. Blazer DG. Depression in late life: Review and commentary. *Journals of Gerontology Series A: Biological Sciences and Medical Sciences* 2003; **58**(3):249–65.

32. Fiske A, Wetherell JL, Gatz M. Depression in older adults. *Annual Review of Clinical Psychology* 2009; **5**:363–89.

33. Blazer DG, Sachs-Ericsson N, Hybels CF. Perception of unmet basic needs as a predictor of depressive symptoms among community-dwelling older adults. *Journal of Gerontology Series A: Biological Sciences and Medical Sciences* 2007; **62**(2):191–5.

34. Hancock GA, Woods B, Challis D, Orrell M. The needs of older people with dementia in residential care. *International Journal of Geriatric Psychiatry* 2006; **21**(1):43–9.

35. van der Ploeg ES, Bax D, Boorsma M, et al. A cross-sectional study to compare care needs of individuals with and without dementia in residential homes in the Netherlands. *BMC Geriatrics* 2013; **13**:1–8.

36. Bakker C, Vugt ME de, van Vliet D, Verhey FRJ, et al. The relationship between unmet care needs in young-onset dementia and the course of neuropsychiatric symptoms: A two-year follow-up study. *International Psychogeriatrics* 2014; **26**(12): 1991–2000.

37. Orrell M, Hancock GA, Liyanage KCG, et al. The needs of people with dementia in care homes: The perspectives of users, staff and family caregivers. *International Psychogeriatrics* 2008; **20**(5):941–51.

38. Kaiser G, Unger A, Marquart B, et al. Die Erfassung des Bedarfs bei Demenzkranken mittels Camberwell Assessment of Need (CANE) for the Elderly. *Neuropsychiatrics* 2010; **24**(3):182–9.

39. Galeone F, Pappalardo S, Chieffi S, et al. Anosognosia for memory deficit in amnestic mild cognitive impairment and Alzheimer's disease. *International Journal of Geriatric Psychiatry* 2011; **26**(7):695–701.

40. Mak E, Chin R, Ng LT, et al. Clinical associations of anosognosia in mild cognitive impairment and Alzheimer's disease. *International Journal of Geriatric Psychiatry* 2015; **30**(12):1207–14.

41. Levinson W, Lesser CS, Epstein RM. Developing physician communication skills for patient-centered care. *Health Affairs (Millwood)* 2010; **29**(7):1310–18.

42. Schäfer I, Hansen H, Schön G, et al. The German MultiCare Study: Patterns of multimorbidity in primary health care—Protocol of a prospective cohort study. *BMC Health Services Research* 2009; **9**:1–9.

43. Iliffe S, Lenihan P, Orrell M, et al. The development of a short instrument to identify common unmet needs in older people in general practice. *British Journal of General Practice* 2004; **54**(509):914–18.

44. Balsinha C, Marques MJ, Gonçalves-Pereira M. A brief assessment unravels unmet needs of older people in primary care: A mixed-methods evaluation of the SPICE tool in Portugal. *Primary Health Care Research & Development* 2018; **19**(6): 637–43.

Unmet Needs of Older Persons with and Without Depression in Residential Homes

Hein van Hout, Jannicke M. Iversen and Marijke Boorsma

4.1 Introduction

Depression is a common disorder in older people and is known to be associated with adverse outcomes such as reduced quality of life and increased morbidity and mortality.[1,2] Among older people in primary care, the prognosis of late-life depression is poor.[3] The prevalence for major depression in residential homes is estimated to be between 6% and 11% and around 30% for depressive symptoms.[4]

There is public pressure on healthcare services to become more responsive to patients' needs. In such a context, needs assessment and detection of unmet needs are considered crucial. 'Need' can be defined as a state where help (or more help) with specific difficulties is required according to care professionals taking the views of the persons themselves into account. An 'unmet' need is defined as a problem for which the participant perceives inappropriate help.[5]

Depressive symptoms seem to be associated with higher rates of unmet needs such as daytime activities, psychological distress, company, memory and communication problems in community-dwelling elderly.[6] The majority of older people and their family carers sampled in general practices in London did not seek help for their unmet needs.[7] To our knowledge, very little is known about the needs of older residents with or without depressive disorders. Greater understanding of health needs for those who are depressed in residential homes will enhance efforts at targeted interventions.

In our study, we hypothesised that (1) persons with depressive disorders in residential homes are less motivated to address their health needs and, for this reason, show more unmet health needs, and (2) the total number of unmet health needs of depressed persons is lower than for those not depressed. Therefore, the aim of this study was to compare the type and number of met and unmet needs among people 65 years of age and older with and without a depressive disorder living in residential homes.

4.2 Methods

4.2.1 Design and Setting

This ancillary study is a part of the Preventive Effects of Disease Management on Disabled Persons Within Homes for Older People (PIKOV) trial.[8] The data described in this study were cross-sectional baseline measurements and involved 11 residential homes of one home care organisation in the northwest of the Netherlands. All mentally competent residents were invited to participate and screened for eligibility. For people lacking in mental capacity, a close family member was approached to provide a proxy report. Lack of mental capacity was a concern for all residents who had dementia. People were included if they were aged 65 years or older, living in a residential home and could respond appropriately to relevant questions. Exclusion criteria were terminal illness and (planned or temporary) referral to a nursing home. Participation was voluntary, and each participant signed a written consent form. The medical ethical committee of the Vrije University Medical Centre approved the study. The sample flowchart is showed in Figure 4.1.

4.2.2 Sampling Procedure

Of the 346 residents, 213 people (58.5%) were approached and interviewed by trained and monthly supervised interviewers. Non-participation at the study was due to refusal of informed consent, terminal illness, inability to complete the interview, age younger than 65 years, incomplete demographical data, incomplete answers on the Primary Care Evaluation of Mental Disorders (PRIME-MD) or an incomplete Camberwell Assessment of Need for the Elderly (CANE) interview.

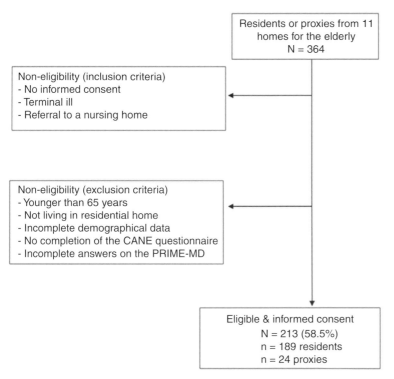

Figure 4.1 Sample derivation

4.2.3   Measures and Measurements

4.2.3.1   Needs Assessment

The CANE instrument was used to assess met and unmet needs. This semi-structured interview has been used in several studies.[6,7,9] It covers 24 areas, including social, physical, psychological and environmental needs; within each area, need was rated as no need, met need or unmet need. A met need was recorded when the participant identified a problem but perceived the available help appropriate to meet the need. An unmet need was recorded when the participant identified a problem but perceived help to be inappropriate or absent. The total numbers of needs, met needs and unmet needs within all areas were recorded. The CANE has shown acceptable psychometric properties.[10,11] The interviews were conducted by trained interviewers and took between 30 and 45 minutes to complete.

4.2.3.2   Major Depressive Disorder

Major depressive disorder was defined in two ways: (1) a diagnosis made by the residents' primary care physician (PCP) or (2) if symptoms met the *Diagnostic and Statistical Manual of Mental Disorders*, 4th edition,

Text Revision (DSM-IV) criteria for major depressive disorder according to the PRIME-MD.[12] The latter was demonstrated to be reliable for identifying major depressive disorders.[13]

4.2.3.3   Potential Confounders and Effect Modifications

The following variables were explored as potential confounders or effect modifications:

Demographical variables: Age and gender of the resident and whether a close family member carried out a proxy interview.

Chronic diseases: For this study, we used the presence and absence of 22 chronic diseases based on the medical records and registered according to the format of the Resident Assessment Instrument Long Term Care Facility (interRAI LTCF).[14] These included, among others, dementia, stroke, cancer, diabetes and cardiovascular diseases.

Activities of daily living: The Groningen Activity Restriction Scale (GARS) is an easy-to-administer, comprehensive measure for assessing disability. Items refer both to activities of daily living (ADLs) and instrumental activities of daily living (IADLs).

An overall score of the 18 items was calculated. The minimum is 18, indicating absence of disability, and the maximum is 72, indicating that a person is highly restricted. This instrument has shown acceptable reliability and validity.[15]

4.2.4 Statistical Analyses

Descriptive statistics (mean, standard deviation and percentages), a t-test and bivariate analyses were calculated for description of the study population (see Table 4.1). Bivariate analyses were also performed to describe met and unmet needs (measured by CANE) among the total group of persons in residential homes (n =213) (see Table 4.3).

Binary logistic regression analyses were performed to compare needs measured by CANE for people who have major depression with non-depressed residents (see Table 4.3), and odds ratios (ORs) with 95% confidence intervals (CIs) were generated. Multiple logistic regression analyses were adjusted for confounders (i.e., age, gender, proxy, GARS and chronic diseases [one or two versus two or more]) to compare needs measured by CANE among people who are depressed or non-depressed (see Table 4.4). We considered confounding to be present when the unadjusted OR changed by 10% or more after adding a variable. Logistic regression analyses were also carried out to explore effect modifications by interaction of the presence of depression

Table 4.1 Description of the Total Study Population (n = 213) and for Persons Who Are Depressed or Non-depressed

Characteristic	Total (n = 213)	Depressed (n = 24)	Non-depressed (n = 189)	OR (CI)[a]	p-Value[b]
Proxy interviewed, n (%)	24 (11.3)	6 (25.0)	18 (9.5)	3.2 (1.1–9.0)	0.024
Gender, n (%)					
Female	158 (74.2)	20 (83.3)	138 (73.0)	1.8 (0.6–5.7)	0.283
Age, mean M (SD)	86.3 (5.2)	85.3 (4.6)	86.4 (5.3)	1.0 (0.9–1.0)	0.318
Age, n (%)[c]					
70–79	23 (10.8)	3 (12.5)	20 (10.6)		
80–89	140 (65.7)	18 (75.0)	122 (64.6)		
>90	50 (23.5)	3 (12.5)	47 (24.9)		
Marital status, n (%)[c]					
Married/ cohabitation	45 (21.1)	3 (12.5)	42 (22.2)		
Single and never been married	18 (8.5)	1 (4.2)	17 (9.0)		
Divorced	4 (1.9)	1 (4.2)	3 (1.6)		
Widowed	146 (68.6)	19 (79.2)	127 (67.2)		
Education, n (%)[c]					
Low	174 (86.1)	23 (95.8)	151 (84.8)		
Middle	21 (10.4)	1 (4.2)	20 (11.2)		
High	7 (3.5)	0 (0.0)	7 (3.9)		
Body mass index (BMI), M (SD)	26.0 (4.7)	27.0 (6.1)	25.9 (4.5)	1.0 (0.8–1.2)	0.336
ADL score, M (SD) (Groningen Activity Restriction Scale)	43.2 (13.3)	40.7 (11.2)	43.5 (13.5)	0.9 (0.9–1.0)	0.072
Chronic diseases, n (%)					
None or one chronic disease	106 (49.8)	15 (62.5)	91 (48.1)	Ref	
Two more chronic diseases	107 (50.2	9 (37.5)	98 (51.9)	0.6 (0.2–1.4)	0.185

[a] Binary logistic regression analyses were used to generate odds ratios (ORs) for independent correlates that were associated with persons who were depressed versus non-depressed.

[b] p-Value for comparing the groups: depressed versus non-depressed.

[c] OR could not be calculated due to insufficiently spread data.

Table 4.2 Total Needs and Respectively Met and Unmet Needs (CANE) Separately for the Total Group of Persons in Residential Homes (*n* = 213)

Item	Total Needs		Met Needs		Unmet Needs	
	n	%	n	%	n	%
Looking after the home	208	97.7	205	98.6	3	1.4
Food	201	94.8	197	98.0	4	2.0
Mobility/falls	195	92.0	185	84.9	10	5.1
Accommodation	164	77.0	163	99.4	1	0.6
Physical illness	158	74.5	158	100.0	0	0.0
Self-care	157	74.4	156	99.4	1	0.6
Managing money	126	59.4	119	94.4	7	5.6
Medication	85	40.3	85	100.0	0	0.0
Incontinence	72	34.3	71	98.6	1	1.4
Eyesight/hearing impairment	71	34.3	59	83.1	12	16.9
Daytime activities	45	21.4	40	88.9	5	11.1
Memory problems	44	21.1	39	88.6	5	11.4
Benefits	31	15.0	30	96.8	1	3.2
Company	21	10.0	13	61.9	8	38.1
Inadvertent self-harm	11	5.2	11	100.0	0	0.0
Caring for someone else	10	4.7	8	80.0	2	20.0
Psychological distress	10	4.8	5	50.0	5	50.0
Information on condition	9	4.3	6	66.7	3	33.3
Psychotic symptoms	4	1.9	2	50.0	2	50.0
Intimate relationships	2	0.9	2	100.0	0	0.0
Abuse/neglect	1	0.5	0	0	1	100.0
Behaviour	1	0.5	1	100.0	0	0.0
Deliberate self-harm	0	0.0	0	0	0	0.0
Alcohol	0	0.0	0	0	0	0.0

with socio-demographic and clinical variables. We did not perform logistical regression analyses if data were insufficiently spread or the numbers were small. SPSS v16.0 was used. Statistical significance was assessed at the $p < 0.05$ level.

4.3 Results

4.3.1 Description of the Study Population

Among the 213 residents participating in this study, a proportion of 11.3% (*n* = 24) of the participants had a depressive disorder. In 3.3% (*n* = 7) of the participants, depression was diagnosed by the GP; in 8.5% (*n* = 18), the symptoms met the DSM-IV criteria for a depressive disorder according to the PRIME-MD, and 0.5% (*n* =

1) was diagnosed by both criteria. Interviews carried out by proxies were significantly more often associated with those diagnosed with depression (25% [*n* = 6] and 9.5% [*n* = 18]; *p* = 0.024) (Table 4.1).

In the total study population, 158 respondents (74.2%) were female (Table 4.1). Mean age of participants was 86.3 years (standard deviation [SD] 5.2 years). Age ranged from 72 to 100 years, and approximately two-thirds of the residents were between 80 and 89 years of age. Over two-thirds of the residents were widowed. The proportion with low education was 86.1%. Mean body mass index (BMI) was 26.0 (SD 4.7) (kg/m^2), and 16% were in the obese range (BMI > 30). Mean total ADL score measured by GARS was 43.2 (SD 13.3), and scores ranged from 18 to 68. Approximately half the respondents had two or more chronic diseases. Most frequently reported were arthrosis (39.4%), myocardial infarction (31.0) and diabetes mellitus (21.1%). These were not differently distributed between depressed and non-depressed persons. There were no significant differences between groups for demographical or clinical variables.

4.3.2 Detecting Confounders and Effect Modifiers

Age, gender, proxy interview, reporting two or more chronic diseases (versus none or one) and GARS were found to confound the differences in needs between depressed and non-depressed persons in 4, 6, 18, 3 and 11 needs, respectively. Proxy interview and GARS were the most frequently confounding variables, meaning that there was a difference in outcome if the interview was completed by the proxy (versus the resident themself) and if the resident had two or more chronic diseases (versus none or one). Therefore, we decided to adjust the analyses in Table 4.3 for these variables. There was only one variable that modified the effect of needs in depressed versus non-depressed persons. Interviews carried out by proxies were significantly more often associated with those diagnosed with depression. A proxy interview modified the need eyesight/hearing impairment, meaning that proxies reported higher number of needs for eyesight/hearing impairment than the residents themselves.

4.3.3 Number and Type of Needs

The average number of identified needs was 7.2 (SD 2.3, range 1–14), and an average of 0.3 (SD 0.9) needs were unmet (range 0–7). In total, 173 (81.2%) persons did not report unmet needs. Of the persons who reported unmet needs ($n = 39$), the mean of unmet needs was 1.8 (SD 1.4, range 1–7). There were 24 people with one unmet need and 15 people with two or more unmet needs.

The needs for the total group of participants in residential homes are described in Table 4.2. The most frequently identified needs (met and unmet together) for the total population were looking after the home (98%), food (95%) and mobility/falls (92%). The needs looking after the home and food were mostly met, but for mobility/falls less frequently. There were no needs reported in the categories alcohol and deliberate self-harm. The most frequently unmet categories were eyesight/hearing impairment (6%), mobility/falls (5%) and company (4%). Although infrequently reported, for the

following categories, people reported relatively many unmet needs: abuse/neglect (100% unmet), psychotic symptoms (50% unmet), psychological distress (50% unmet), company (38% unmet) and information on condition (33% unmet).

4.3.4 Needs of Persons with and Without Depression

There was no significant difference in the total number of needs reported by depressed persons and those reported by non-depressed persons (respectively, 8.1 versus 7.1 needs). However, the number of participants who reported 10 or more needs was 50% in depressed people ($n = 2$) and 32% ($n = 7$) in those not depressed. Among those depressed, the needs looking after the home (100%), food (100%) and mobility/falls (96%) were most often reported.

Bivariate logistic regression analyses showed that the needs daytime activities, company, psychological distress, psychotic symptoms, medication and benefits were more prevalent among people who were depressed (Table 4.3). However, in the adjusted analyses, the differences in medication and benefits did not remain significant. Finally, those depressed were more likely to report needs in relation to daytime activities (OR = 3.1; CI 1.0–9.5), company (OR = 3.7; CI 1.1–21.1), psychological distress (OR = 13.3; CI 2.9–61.9) and psychotic symptoms (OR = 11.7; CI 1.4–94.7) (Table 4.3).

Both depressed and non-depressed older people showed few unmet needs. Categories with most frequently identified unmet needs in depressed residents were company (16.7%), eyesight/hearing impairment (12.5%), mobility/falls (12.5%) and psychological distress (12.5%) (Figure 4.2).

In total, 71% of depressed persons and 83% of non-depressed persons reported no unmet needs at all. Depressed people reported more total unmet needs than non-depressed people (0.9 [SD 1.9] versus 0.3 [SD 0.7], $p = 0.009$). Of the people who reported at least one unmet need, the mean number of unmet needs for depressed people was 3.0 (SD 2.5) versus 1.5 (SD 0.8) for those who were non-depressed ($p = 0.037$) (Table 4.4).

4.4 Discussion

4.4.1 Main Results

Participants who were depressed were more likely to report needs in relation to daytime activities, company,

Table 4.3 Needs Measured by CANE Among Persons Who Are Depressed or Non-depressed

Need	Depressed, n (%) (n = 24)	Non-depressed, n (%) (n = 189)	OR (CI),[a] Unadjusted	p-Value[b]	OR (CI),[c] Adjusted	p-Value[d]
Looking after the home	24 (100.0)	184 (97.4)	[e]		[e]	
Food	23 (100.0)	178 (94.2)	[e]		[e]	
Mobility/falls	23 (95.8)	172 (91.5)	2.1 (0.3–16.9)		[e]	
Self-care	19 (82.6)	138 (73.4)	1.7 (0.6–5.3)		1.0 (0.2–3.9)	
Physical illness	18 (75.0)	140 (74.5)	1.0 (0.4–2.7)		1.1 (0.3–3.4)	
Managing money	18 (75.0)	108 (57.4)	2.2 (0.8–5.9)		1.4 (0.5–4.0)	
Accommodation	15 (62.5)	149 (78.8)	0.4 (0.2–1.1)		0.4 (0.1–1.1)	
Medication	15 (65.2)	70 (37.2)	3.2 (1.3–7.8)	0.013	2.3 (0.8–6.5)	
Daytime activities	10 (43.5)	35 (18.7)	3.3 (1.4–8.3)	0.009	3.1 (1.0–9.5)	0.044
Eyesight/hearing impairment	9 (37.5)	62 (33.9)	1.2 (0.5–2.8)		1.2 (0.4–3.1)	
Benefits	8 (33.3)	23 (12.6)	3.5 (1.3–9.0)	0.011	1.6 (0.4–6.4)	
Company	7 (29.2)	14 (7.6)	5.0 (1.8–14.2)	0.002	3.7 (1.1–21.1)	0.029
Memory problems	7 (30.4)	37 (19.9)	1.8 (0.7–4.6)		0.8 (0.2–2.9)	
Incontinence	6 (25.0)	66 (35.5)	0.6 (0.2–1.6)		0.4 (0.1–1.1)	
Psychological distress	6 (26.1)	4 (2.2)	15.9 (4.1–61.8)	<0.001	13.3 (2.9–61.9)	0.001
Information on condition	4 (17.4)	5 (2.7)	7.7 (1.9–31.0)	0.004	4.2 (0.8–23.0)	
Psychotic symptoms	2 (8.3)	2 (1.1)	8.3 (1.1–61.7)	0.039	11.7 (1.4–94.7)	0.021
Inadvertent self-harm	2 (8.3)	9 (4.8)	1.8 (0.4–8.9)		0.9 (0.2–5.4)	
Caring for someone else	1 (4.2)	9 (4.8)	0.9 (0.1–7.1)		1.7 (0.2–15.5)	
Deliberate self-harm	0 (0.0)	0 (0.0)	[e]		[e]	
Abuse/neglect	0 (0.0)	1 (0.5)	[e]		[e]	
Behaviour	0 (0.0)	1 (0.5)	[e]		[e]	
Alcohol	0 (0.0)	0 (0.0)	[e]		[e]	
Intimate relationships	0 (0.0)	2 (1.1)	[e]		[e]	
Total needs, M (SD)	8.1 (2.5)	7.1 (2.2)	1.2 (1.0–1.4)		1.1 (0.8–1.5)	

[a] Unadjusted logistic regression was used to generate the odds ratios (OR) for independent correlates associated with persons who were depressed versus non-depressed.

[b] p < 0.05 for unadjusted analyses.

[c] Logistic regression adjusted for age, gender, proxy, chronic diseases and ADL (GARS) was used to generate ORs.

[d] p < 0.05 for adjusted analyses.

[e] Could not be calculated due to insufficiently spread data.

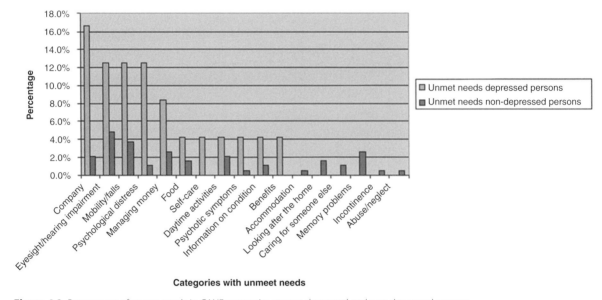

Figure 4.2 Percentages of unmet needs in CANE categories among depressed and non-depressed persons

psychological distress and psychotic symptoms. Both depressed and non-depressed older people showed few unmet needs. However, depressed people reported more total unmet needs than non-depressed people.

4.4.2 Discussion of Results

In this sample of depressed people, the numbers of unmet needs were very low. It is possible that older people based their needs on the care they thought was available. By contrast, it is possible that the care in the participating residential homes was responsive to the persons' expressed needs and that appropriate care was provided to them.

The total number of needs found in our study was relatively low. It is possible that our population was less disabled than the population with dementia described earlier by Hancock et al.[6] Alternatively, this could be due to the fact that the number of needs in some other studies is the average of the reported needs by residents, staff and sometimes the carers together. Hancock et al.[6] found that depressed residents with dementia have higher rates of unmet needs than those without dementia. Despite the few numbers of unmet needs among participants with depression without dementia, depressed people in our study reported more total unmet needs than non-depressed people. This emphasises that depressed people in residential homes, irrespective of dementia, are vulnerable and need special attention.

In this study, depressed people were more likely to report unmet social needs (daytime activities or company). This is in accordance with a study among residents in homes for older people, where it was reported that those who were depressed undertook little social activity and were visited infrequently.[16] In a study among people with dementia, depression was associated with higher rates of unmet social needs.[6] Our results emphasise the need for more adequate treatment related to social needs among depressed older patients. Walters et al.[7] conclude that the majority of older people and their carers do not seek help for their unmet needs, and this is for several reasons: a low motivation to seek help (with a strong sense of resignation, withdrawal and low expectations) and a tendency to minimise problems or relate them to their age.

In this study, depressed people were also more likely to report needs related to mental health as psychotic symptoms and psychological distress. We need to be very cautious about interpreting these results because these needs had very large confidence intervals and concerned very few people.

Depression in older persons is often untreated and can be persistent.[3] Therefore, it is important to identify people at high risk of having or developing depression. Furthermore, early interventions in residential homes can positively influence depressive symptoms.[17] Bagley et al.[18] highlight that despite the high prevalence rate of depression, recognition of depression in newly admitted residents by staff members was limited. Therefore, older people who are newly admitted to long-term care facilities need more attention, particularly with regard to

Table 4.4 Unmet Needs (CANE) Among Persons Who Are Depressed or Non-depressed

Unmet Need	Depressed, n (%) (n = 24)	Non-depressed, n (%) (n = 189)	OR (CI)[a]	p-Value[b]
Company	4 (16.7)	4 (2.1)	9.3 (2.1–39.9)	<0.001
Eyesight/hearing impairment	3 (12.5)	9 (4.8)	2.9 (0.7–11.4)	0.121
Mobility/falls	3 (12.5)	7 (3.7)	3.7 (0.9–15.5)	0.055
Psychological distress	3 (12.5)	2 (1.1)	13.4 (2.1–84.5)	<0.001
Managing money	2 (8.3)	5 (2.6)	3.3 (0.6–18.3)	0.141
Food	1 (4.2)	3 (1.6)	2.7 (0.3–27)	0.381
Self-care	1 (4.2)	0 (0.0)	[c]	
Daytime activities	1 (4.2)	4 (2.1)	2.0 (0.2–18.8)	0.532
Psychotic symptoms	1 (4.2)	1 (0.5)	8.2 (0.5–135.1)	0.082
Information on condition	1 (4.2)	2 (1.1)	4.1 (0.4–46.6)	0.223
Benefits	1 (4.2)	0 (0.0)	[c]	
Accommodation	0 (0.0)	1 (0.5)	[c]	
Looking after the home	0 (0.0)	3 (1.6)	[c]	
Caring for someone else	0 (0.0)	2 (1.1)	[c]	
Memory problems	0 (0.0)	5 (2.6)	[c]	
Incontinence	0 (0.0)	1 (0.5)	[c]	
Physical illness	0 (0.0)	0 (0.0)	[c]	
Medication	0 (0.0)	0 (0.0)	[c]	
Deliberate self-harm	0 (0.0)	0 (0.0)	[c]	
Inadvertent self-harm	0 (0.0)	0 (0.0)	[c]	
Abuse/neglect	0 (0.0)	1 (0.5)	[c]	
Behaviour	0 (0.0)	0 (0.0)	[c]	
Alcohol	0 (0.0)	0 (0.0)	[c]	
Intimate relationships	0 (0.0)	0 (0.0)	[c]	
Total unmet needs, M (SD)	0.9 (1.9)	0.3 (0.7)	1.6 (1.1–2.3)	0.009
Total unmet needs among persons with at least one unmet need, mean M (SD)	3.0 (2.5)	1.5 (0.8)	1.9 (1.0–3.5)	0.037

[a] Unadjusted logistic regression was used to generate odds ratios (ORs) for independent correlates associated with persons who were depressed versus non-depressed.

[b] p < 0.05 for unadjusted analyses.

[c] ORs and p-values could not be calculated due to small number of groups (<5).

depression. In order to improve mental health care, it is important to identify patients at high risk of persistent depression.[19] Meeting their psychosocial needs better may also contribute to reducing the depressive symptoms of residents in residential homes.

1.4.3 Strengths and Limitations

This study measured needs in a large, virtually unselected sample of older residents. It was a strength of the study that depression was diagnosed in two ways, either by a diagnosis from the GP or by symptoms of depression in accordance with DSM-IV criteria. By contrast, those who were diagnosed by their GP did not appear to have symptoms at the time of the measurement and were possibly different or in remission compared to those diagnosed in accordance with DSM-IV criteria. It is therefore possible that we have included patients with emotional distress or a possible case of depression as actually having depression. Furthermore, it is also possible that we have underestimated the number of people with depression because non-participation may be a consequence of their depression. Interviews carried out by proxies were significantly more often associated with those diagnosed with depression. However, this seems to be a general problem in other studies as well.[6] A limitation of using interviews to obtain data in depressed persons in long-term care is that they are less capable of addressing their health needs and therefore report fewer health needs, both met and unmet. In the ORs presented, there were large confidence intervals, which means that this concerned few people. Psychological distress and psychotic symptoms needs were more likely in those depressed than in those non-depressed. This may not be surprising because depression, psychological distress and, in a limited way, also psychotic symptoms are related concepts. Despite these limitations, this study provides a reasonable representation of the proportion of met and unmet health needs of persons with and without depression living in residential homes in the Netherlands.

4.5 Conclusion

Our study showed low numbers of unmet needs in older people living in residential homes. However, depressed people were more likely to report more unmet needs in total. Therefore, healthcare personnel need to be cautious to better meet the needs of depressed persons. Possible intervention strategies for depressive residents may focus on specific needs such as more daytime activities and company.

Acknowledgements

Recruitment and data collection were made available by grants from the Netherlands Organisation for Health Research and Development (ZonMw Grant No. 945–05-030).

References

1. Cuijpers P, Smit F. Excess mortality in depression: A meta-analysis of community studies. *Journal of Affective Disorders* 2002; **72**(3):227–36.

2. Licht-Strunk E, van der Kooij KG, van Schaik DJ, et al. Prevalence of depression in older patients consulting their general practitioner in the Netherlands. *International Journal of Geriatric Psychiatry: A Journal of the Psychiatry of Late Life and Allied Sciences* 2005; **20**(11):1013–19.

3. Licht-Strunk E, Beekman AT, de Haan M, van Marwijk HW. The prognosis of undetected depression in older general practice patients: A one year follow-up study. *Journal of Affective Disorders* 2009; **114**(1–3):310–15.

4. Eisses AM, Kluiter H, Jongenelis K, et al. Risk indicators of depression in residential homes. *International Journal of Geriatric Psychiatry* 2004; **19** (7):634–40.

5. van Hout H, Droes RM, van der Ploeg ES. *Camberwell's Assessment of Needs in the Elderly (CANE): Dutch Manual*. Amsterdam: VUmc, EMGO Instituut; 2001.

6. Hancock GA, Woods B, Challis D, Orrell M. The needs of older people with dementia in residential care. *International Journal of Geriatric Psychiatry: A Journal of the Psychiatry of Late Life and Allied Sciences* 2006; **21**(1):43–9.

7. Walters K, Iliffe S, Orrell M. An exploration of help-seeking behaviour in older people with unmet needs. *Family Practice* 2001; **18**(3):277–82.

8. Boorsma M, van Hout HP, Frijters DH, et al. The cost-effectiveness of a new disease management model for frail elderly living in homes for the elderly: Design of a cluster randomized, controlled clinical trial. *BMC Health Services Research* 2008; **8**(1):1–7.

9. Walters K, Iliffe S, Tai SS, Orrell M. Assessing needs from patient, carer and professional perspectives: The Camberwell Assessment of Need for Elderly people in primary care. *Age & Ageing* 2000; **29**(6):505–10.

10. van der Roest HG, Meiland FJ, van Hout HP, et al. Validity and reliability of the Dutch version of the Camberwell Assessment of Need for the Elderly in community-dwelling people with dementia. *International Psychogeriatrics* 2008; **20**(6):1273–90.

11. Reynolds T, Thornicroft G, Abas M, et al. Camberwell Assessment of Need for the Elderly (CANE): Development, validity and reliability. *British Journal of Psychiatry* 2000; **176**(5):444–52.

12. Spitzer RL, Kroenke K, Williams JB, Patient Health Questionnaire Primary Care Study Group: Validation and utility of a self-report version of PRIME-MD: The PHQ primary care study. *Journal of the American Medical Association* 1999; **282**(18):1737–44.

13. Bakker IM, Terluin B, van Marwijk HW, et al. Test–retest reliability of the PRIME-MD: Limitations in diagnosing mental disorders in primary care. *European Journal of Public Health* 2009; **19**(3):303–7.

14. interRAI LTCF. Long-Term Care Facility; available at www.interrai.org.

15. Kempen GI, Miedema I, Ormel J, Molenaar W. The assessment of disability with the Groningen Activity Restriction Scale: Conceptual framework and

psychometric properties. *Social Science & Medicine* 1996; **43**(11):1601–10.

16. Ames D. Depression among elderly residents of local-authority residential homes. *British Journal of Psychiatry* 1990; **156**(5):667–75.

17. Cuijpers P, Lammeren PV. Secondary prevention of depressive symptoms in elderly inhabitants of residential homes. *International Journal of Geriatric Psychiatry* 2001; **16**(7):702–8.

18. Bagley H, Cordingley L, Burns A, et al. Recognition of depression by staff in nursing and residential homes. *Journal of Clinical Nursing* 2000; **9**(3):445–50.

19. Licht-Strunk E, van der Windt DA, Van Marwijk HW, et al. The prognosis of depression in older patients in general practice and the community: A systematic review. *Family Practice* 2007; **24**(2): 168–80.

Chapter

5

Needs of Older People Living Alone
A Critical Review

Raffaela Carvacho and Claudia Miranda-Castillo

5.1 Introduction

In a rapidly ageing world, more and more older people live alone.[1] Whereas almost one-third of the older adult population in the United States lives alone,[2] more than 50% of those over age 75 in the United Kingdom live by themselves.[3] Although this phenomenon varies widely throughout the world (mainly observed in developed countries), its social relevance and study have increased in recent decades.[4] In general terms, older people who live alone tend to be elderly women, widowed spouses, have a higher level of education and tend to use health services more often than those who live accompanied.[1,4–6] Nevertheless, the amount of information available about this population is still sparse. On the one hand, the increase in those who live alone is positive, given that the majority of older people want to age in place and maintain their independence and autonomy as long as possible,[7] but, on the other hand, according to the World Health Organization,[8] older people living alone are also considered a risk group that should be targeted by social and preventive health programmes to ensure that they have the necessary resources to meet their needs. For example, for 'younger' older people who are beginning their older adulthood, the availability of financial resources (having savings and good pensions for this stage) largely determines the possibility of living alone; however, as their age increases, their health becomes more relevant in determining that possibility.[4] This means that this population necessarily requires special care of their physical and mental health so that they can retain their autonomy for as long as possible.

Kharicha et al.[9] indicated that older people living alone are at significantly higher risk of functional impairment, falls, poor diet, social isolation and certain diseases (such as arthritis, rheumatism, glaucoma and cataracts), even after having adjusted for variables such as age, sex, income and level of education. Living alone is an especially delicate situation because it implies a risk for falls, events that can drastically transform the state of health and functionality of an older person.[10] Thus, it has been observed that this population has a greater tendency to use emergency departments and see a general practitioner and are also more likely to have mental health conditions. Likewise, another study[11] found that older people who shared a home with their families had better indicators of physical health, self-esteem and health promoting behaviours than those who lived alone. In addition, it has been observed that living alone is significantly associated with an increase in mortality regardless of age, sex, marital status and health status.[12]

Older people living alone can be classified into two groups: those who live alone but receive support from a family carer who visits or calls them regularly and those who live alone without support from an identifiable carer (family or friend). In the first instance, this relative is called a *long-distance carer* and is generally someone who provides informal (unpaid) support to the older person without sharing the same home and who probably does not identify themselves as a carer but rather as 'family'.[13] It is estimated that 15% of family carers could be classed as long-distance carers.[14] It should be noted that there is no consensus on the definition of this role yet, and although it is a growing phenomenon, information about this population, their characteristics and experiences is still scarce.[15] Furthermore, there is even less information about older people living alone without a long-distance carer. In this group, there is a high risk of social isolation, a lack of structural and functional social support and loneliness, resulting in negative perceptions or emotions about their social networks. Both phenomena put older people at high risk of having poor health.[16]

Thus, formal (paid) care providers are called to give special attention to older people living alone seeking to identify their needs in time and effectively meet those needs.[17] Faced with this reality, it becomes relevant to know which needs are apparent and their frequency and distribution and to evaluate them in a comprehensive and multidimensional manner. In this context, the Camberwell Assessment of Need for the Elderly (CANE) can usefully identify various needs that are grouped into different dimensions (e.g., environmental, physical, psychological and social) and differentiate between met and unmet needs. The information this provides may reveal interesting patterns and new opportunities for interventions focused on older people living alone. Therefore, the aim of this chapter is to examine and describe the studies in which the CANE has been applied to older people living alone in order to know their met and unmet needs and to explore the relationship between the latter and their living arrangements.

5.2 Method

5.2.1 Search Strategies

A critical review was performed in August 2019. An overview of the needs of older people living alone according to the CANE and some relationships among those variables highlighted important gaps in research on this topic. The study selection followed the guidelines of the Preferred Reporting Items for Systematic Reviews and Meta-Analyses (PRISMA) flow diagram made by Moher et al.[18] A search of studies published in the last 20 years, in English or Spanish, was carried out on the MEDLINE, SCOPUS and CINHAL databases using the following keywords: 'needs assessment', 'CANE', 'living alone', 'solitary living' and 'older people'.

5.2.2 Inclusion and Exclusion Criteria

The inclusion criteria for the review were empirical, cross-sectional or longitudinal studies that measured needs as a primary or secondary outcome through CANE and included people aged 60 years and above living alone in the community. Studies that did not meet these criteria were excluded, as well as those with mixed samples (people living alone versus accompanied or younger versus older people living alone) without considering separate analyses.

5.3 Results

The initial search yielded 266 titles. Firstly, all duplicate titles were eliminated, resulting in 132 studies. A further five studies were added through screening papers' references. Titles and abstracts were analysed in all 137 studies. Secondly, full texts of the 22 studies that passed the initial screening were analysed. Finally, studies which did not meet the inclusion criteria or did not report all the necessary information were eliminated, resulting in a total of six studies (see Figure 5.1). The two authors of this chapter extracted the relevant information independently and discussed any disagreements. Of the 16 rejected papers, one was excluded because the entire sample lived accompanied, six studies focused on institutionalised populations and three were excluded because they did not report information about living arrangements. A further six were excluded because although significant numbers of the sample lived alone (between 20% and 52%), the analyses were performed for the entire sample without reporting analyses by living arrangements.

As for the studies that were finally selected, there was great heterogeneity in their samples. Two studies focused on outpatients with mental health problems treated in psychiatric settings (including older people with dementia, depression, schizophrenia and delirium)[19,20], another two studies focused on older people with dementia,[21,22] one study addressed an older population without mental health problems who had physical problems,[23] and the last and most recent study comprised a population-representative sample of people older than 75 years for whom the CANE was applied via telephone.[24] For more information, see Table 5.1.

The six selected studies used CANE to identify frequency and areas of met and unmet needs and also analysed which factors acted as predictors of the needs identified. Only one of the studies[21] directly compared older people with dementia living alone (with and without a long-distance family carer) versus those who lived accompanied.

5.3.1 Met and Unmet Needs of People Living Alone

Studies addressing older populations with mental health disorders recruited through mental health and liaison psychiatry services[19,20] showed that older people who lived alone reported significantly fewer met needs (compared to those who lived accompanied), and they had more unmet needs. The areas where they reported significantly more unmet needs

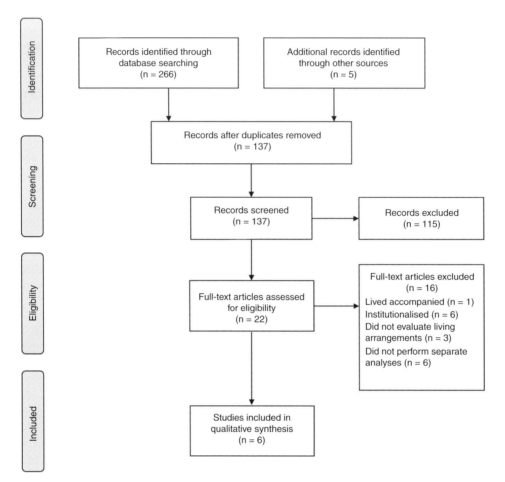

Figure 5.1 Study selection process

were food ($\chi^2 = 6.3$, $p < 0.01$), daytime activities ($\chi^2 = 14.7$, $p < 0.01$) and psychotic symptoms ($\chi^2 = 5.0$, $p < 0.01$).[20] An analysis of variance (ANOVA) test indicated that men had significantly more unmet needs than women with dementia living alone [$F(3, 42) = 3.7$, $p < 0.05$], but gender was not a significant predictor of unmet needs.[20] As for the community-dwelling sample of older people living with dementia, van der Roest et al.[22] found that approximately one-third of them lived alone (36.5%). Their results indicated that people who lived alone reported significantly more met needs (mean [M]= 5.5, standard deviation [SD] = 2.8) than those who lived with their carer ($M = 4.5$, SD = 2.6; $t_{(209)} = -2.67$, $p = 0.01$). It was also observed that informal carers who lived with the person with dementia reported significantly fewer unmet needs for their care recipient ($M = 1.4$, SD = 1.8) compared to those who did not live with the

person with dementia ($M = 2.15$, SD = 2.5; $U = 10,231.00$, $p = 0.03$). A study by Miranda-Castillo et al.[21] focused on met and unmet needs of people with dementia rated by researchers. It was found that people with dementia living alone had a lower number of met needs ($M = 7.1$, SD 3.4, range 1–17) and a higher number of unmet needs ($M = 3.9$, SD 3.1, range 0–11) compared to people with dementia who lived accompanied ($M = 7.5$, SD 2.5, range 2–14 and $M = 2.0$, SD 2.0, range 0–7, respectively). The difference between the met needs of both groups was not significant, whereas the difference between unmet needs was ($p < 0.01$). This study also described the areas where unmet needs of people with dementia who lived alone were most frequent: daily activities (54%), company (52%), psychological distress (44%), eyesight/hearing (32%) and accidental self-harm (32%). In addition, when comparing met and unmet needs in each area

Table 5.1 Characteristics of Selected Studies

Author, Year, Country	Recruitment Context	Health Status	Sample	Met and Unmet Needs
1. Stein et al., 2019, Germany	In the community	Mental health: no cognitive impairment Physical health: not reported	Total n = 845; age M = 80.32 years (SD: 4.56 years); women (58.3%); people living alone = not reported	Reported of the total n: Met needs: M = 9.2 (standard deviation [SD]: not reported). Main areas: not reported Unmet needs: M = 2.0 (SD: not reported) Main areas: memory (n = 62, 7.4%); physical health (n = 58, 6.7%); mobility (n = 56, 6.3%)
2. Hermsen et al., 2017, Netherlands	In the community, primary care	Mental health: no cognitive impairment Physical health: fragility, joint pain and co-morbidity (at least two chronic diseases)	Total n = 407; age M = 76.8 years (SD: 6.3 years); women (62.4%); people living alone = 165 (40.5%)	Reported of the total n: Met needs: M = 3.7 (SD: not reported). Main areas: personal care (100%); medication (97.9%); food (96.8%) Unmet needs: M = 0.3 (SD: 0.8, range: 0–13). Main areas: company (67%); daily activities (37%); caring for another (31%); information (26%)
3. Passos et al., 2017, Portugal	Inpatients (n = 32) and outpatients (n = 274) in a hospital psychiatry unit	Mental health: depression (33.7%), dementia (24.5%), schizophrenia (12.7%) of the sample Physical health: not reported	n = 306; age M = 74 years (SD: 6 years); women (73.9%); people living alone = 53 (17.3%)	Met needs: inpatients (not reported); Outpatients (not reported) Main areas: not reported Unmet needs: inpatients: not reported; outpatients: not reported Main areas: inpatients: daily activities (62.5%), medication (21.9%), psychological distress (40.6%); outpatients: daily activities (44.9%), memory (12.8%), psychological distress (24.1%)
4. Miranda-Castillo et al., 2010, England	Primary or hospital care (memory clinics)	Mental health: dementia Physical health: not reported	People living alone with remote carer = 128; people living alone without a remote carer = 24; age M = 81.7 years (SD: 5.9 years)	Living alone: Met needs: M = 7.1 (SD: 3.4) Main areas: memory (92%), food (70%), money (68%) Unmet needs: M = 3.9 (SD: 3.1) Main areas: daytime activities (27, 54.0%), company (26, 52.0%), psychological distress (22, 44.0%), eyesight/hearing (16, 32.0%), accidental self-harm (16, 32.0%) Living with others Met needs: M = 7.5 (SD: 2.5) Main areas: memory (95.1%), food (86.3%), looking after home (83.3%) Unmet needs: M = 2.0 (SD: 2.0) Main areas: daytime activities (50, 49.0%), company (34, 33.0%), psychological distress (25, 24.5%), eyesight/hearing (17, 16.7%)
5. Greaves et al., 2006, England	Inpatients referred to liaison psychiatry from medical or surgical units	Mental health: dementia (43%), depression (33.3%), delirium (8.8%) Physical health: vascular brain accident (5.4%) Without any psychiatric diagnosis (2.6%)	n = 117 years; age M = 81 years (SD: 6.9 years); women (50.4%)	Reported of the total n: Met needs: M = 2.7 (SD: 2.5) Main areas: physical health (59%), personal care (24.8%), food (24.8%) Unmet needs: M = 4.4 (SD: 2.9) Main areas: memory (49.6%), psychological distress (46.2%), mobility (44.4%)
6. van der Roest et al., 2009, Netherlands	In the community, care in day-care centres or memory clinics	Mental health: dementia diagnosed Physical health: not reported	n = 236; women (54.8%); age M = 79.8 years (SD: 7.6 years)	Reported of the total n: Global needs: M = 9.6 (SD: 3.4); unmet needs: M = 1.7 (SD: not reported) Main areas of unmet needs: daily activities (13.1%), company (60.3%), memory (32.5%)

of the CANE by living arrangement, home care (χ^2 = 17.23, $p < 0.001$), food (χ^2 = 13.91, $p < 0.002$), self-care (χ^2 = 10.23, p < 0.002) and accidental self-harm (χ^2 = 16.51, $p < 0.001$) presented significantly more often as unmet needs in people with dementia living alone.

Regarding predictors of unmet needs in people with dementia living alone, the only predictor was the number of behavioural and psychological symptoms (F_{ANOVA} = 22.4, $p < 0.01$, R^2 = 0.63).[21] In addition, the same study showed that people with dementia who lived alone received significantly more formal services than those who lived accompanied. These services were mainly outpatient (60%), psychiatric (55.2%), general practitioners (53.3%) and home care (45.7%).

Hermsen et al.[23] assessed self-perceived needs of older people with physical morbidity who did not have identified mental health problems. Participants had joint pain and co-morbidity (the latter being understood as the presence of at least two chronic diseases). Approximately 40% of the sample lived alone, and based on a multivariate analysis, a significant association was found between living alone and presenting a greater number of unmet needs in a psychosocial area, such as memory, company, daytime activities and information (odds ratio [OR] = 1.62, 95% confidence interval [CI] = 1.13–2.31, $p < 0.001$). It is worth mentioning that although few older people in the total sample reported needs in the psychosocial area, most of these were unmet, and those who lived alone received less social support or reported more symptoms of depression and were the ones who presented more psychosocial needs. In another study that was based on a population-representative telephone survey for the older population aged 75 years and older with a total sample of 845 individuals,[24] it was found that older people living alone had a significant tendency to develop more symptoms of depression (OR = 1.701, 95% CI = 1.022–2.832, $p = 0.04$), which, in turn, were associated with a higher number of unmet needs (OR = 1.824, 95% CI = 1.532–2.171, $p < 0.001$).

5.4 Discussion

To our knowledge, this is the first review that examines the needs of older people living alone through application of the CANE. According to the results, people living alone tend to have a lower number of met needs and a greater number of unmet needs.[20,21]

This finding is consistent with World Health Organization's statement about older people living alone being identified as a risk group.[8] Similarly, other studies have also found a lack of or insufficient help to reduce or solve a specific difficulty (e.g., health problems, loneliness, self-esteem problems and fall prevention, among others) and a high presence of risk factors in this population.[9,11,12,25,26] It should be noted that the results included in this review came mostly from people who had a mental health problem, especially dementia. Therefore, these results should be viewed with caution, especially in relation to the general population of older people living alone. In addition, not all of the included studies presented results showing the same trend. Van der Roest et al.[22] reported that people with dementia who did not live with their carer reported more met needs than those who did. This could be explained by the difference in coverage that formal services have in different countries. However, van der Roest et al.[22] advised viewing their results with caution given that some older people with dementia living alone were difficult to reach by phone, and many were not included because they could not be contacted.

It is important to point out that living alone is not necessarily harmful, and many older people find living alone to be a positive experience. Some studies have observed increased levels of satisfaction with life, independence in daily life activities,[27] better well-being[28] and better adherence to interventions[10] in older people living alone. In this sense, some authors argue that the key to living well lies in the level of attachment that the older person living alone has to their community, which implies that social support might act as a buffer for the negative aspects associated with living alone.[26,28] In addition, older people living alone and who isolate themselves socially are more likely to experience feelings of loneliness, which, in turn, are detrimental to their health and well-being.[29]

The results of this review suggest the importance of the role played by social support given that the areas that concentrated the greatest number of unmet needs in older people living alone both with and without mental health problems were those of a psychosocial nature, such as daily activities, company and psychological distress.[20–23] This is in line with previous literature about frail older people living alone, who experienced more problems in the psychosocial area: more symptoms of depression, lower levels of life satisfaction and greater social isolation.[30] To this extent, there is clear evidence of the need for generating psychosocial interventions for older people living alone that promote social participation and active aging in both people who have and those who do not have mental health issues.

It is a matter of concern that older people with dementia living alone rarely access formal care on their own. Access to services is usually mediated by an informal carer.[21] This leaves older people who live alone and who have smaller support networks at a greater disadvantage. The same authors[21] stated that needs were covered mainly by the family carer, but it seems that a family care alone is not enough or is not adequate to meet some of the needs. Therefore, access to more formal support services is vital for meeting the needs of older people living alone. In order to achieve this, health professionals and social workers must be able to identify and collaborate with other actors, such as family carers, including long-distance carers. With regard to this, it was found that remote family carers have specific characteristics: they tend to be younger, they are often children and women, they have fewer depressive symptoms, and they report more unmet needs of the person with dementia living alone compared to carers who share the household.[21,22] Either distance prevents the family carer from being adequately informed about the needs of the older person and communication is less effective, or long-distance carers have a bigger perspective and therefore have a greater facility to identify changes or difficult situations compared to family carers who share the home with the older person. More research is needed about the characteristics and needs of long-distance family carers because they can be key actors in collaboration with formal care services.[31]

5.4.1 Future Research

It is worth mentioning that the variable living alone was barely addressed in needs assessment research, especially considering that this population comprised a third or even half of some of the samples in the included studies. These articles only described the variable but did not report any analysis associated with living arrangement. It is not clear whether these studies did not actually perform analyses around the variable of interest or if results were not reported because they were not significant (reporting bias).

Because this is a hard to reach population, researching the needs of older people living alone (and especially those with dementia) is difficult to carry out. Therefore, this is a major challenge for future research in ageing and needs. In summary, more research is needed regarding met and unmet needs of older people living alone, covering different types of populations, such as those with and without mental health issues and those with and without long-distance carers.

5.4.2 Limitations

One of the strengths of this review is related to the homogeneity in the concept of needs addressed through the CANE, which has good psychometric properties and was validated for most of the samples evaluated. However, this review had several limitations. Only a few studies met the inclusion and exclusion criteria. In addition, all selected studies had a cross-sectional design and small samples, so causal relationships between the reviewed factors could not be considered. Furthermore, the samples did not necessarily represent the diversity of older people living alone in the community, which prevents conclusive results from being drawn by the results of this review. Finally, some relevant data about needs were not reported for the subsample of older people living alone, and consequently, no further information could be extracted.

5.5 Conclusion

Little is known about met and unmet needs of older people living alone in the community. Research using the CANE has yielded more information about met and unmet needs of older people living alone with dementia rather than any other group of older people living alone. It has been found that this particular group has a lower number of met needs and a higher number of unmet needs compared to those living with others. Finally, the identified unmet needs were most commonly found in the psychosocial domain.

Even though living alone can be a positive experience and a voluntary choice for many older people, it can also be a risk factor for social isolation, mental health problems and loneliness. Therefore, it is essential that we move forward in understanding the needs of older people living alone, which could lead to developing more adequate and person-centred interventions in collaboration with key actors from both informal (unpaid family care) and formal sources of support.

Acknowledgements

This work was supported by the Vicerrectoría of Research, Pontificia Universidad Católica de Chile (Grant INTERDISCIPLINA II170053), by the National Agency for Research and Development (ANID), FONDECYT (Grant 1191726) and by the Fund for Innovation and Competitiveness (FIC) of the Chilean Ministry of Economy, Development and Tourism through the Millennium Science Initiative (Grant IS130005); all grants were awarded to Claudia Miranda-Castillo. Raffaela Carvacho was supported by the National Commission for Scientific and Technological Development (CONICYT) Scholarship for studying master programmes and Vicerrectoría of Research, Pontificia Universidad Católica de Chile (Grant INTERDISCIPLINA II170053).

References

1. Department of Economic and Social Affairs. Living arrangements of older persons: A report on an expanded international dataset. United Nations, New York, 2017. Available at www.un.org/en/development/desa/population/publications/pdf/ageing/LivingArrangements.pdf.

2. Federal Interagency Forum on Aging-Related Statistics. Older Americans 2010: Key indicators of well-being. Department of Health and Human Services, Washington, DC, 2010. Available at https://agingstats.gov/docs/PastReports/2010/OA2010.pdf.

3. Office for National Statistics. General Household Survey 2007. UK Statistics Authority, London, January 2009. Available at https://webarchive.nationalarchives.gov.uk/20160115215936 or www.ons.gov.uk/ons/publications/re-reference-tables.html?edition=tcmpercent3A77-53869.

4. Reher D, Requena M. Living alone in later life: A global perspective. *Population and Development Review* 2018; **44**(3):427–54.

5. Age UK. Later life in the United Kingdom. London, May 2019. Available at www.ageuk.org.uk/globalassets/age-uk/documents/reports-and-publications/later_life_uk_factsheet.pdf.

6. Dreyer K, Steventon A, Fisher R, Deeny SR. The association between living alone and health care utilisation in older adults: A retrospective cohort study of electronic health records from a London general practice. *BMC Geriatrics* 2018; **18**:15–17.

7. Lecovich E. Aging in place: From theory to practice. *Anthropological Notebooks* 2014; **20**(1):21–32.

8. World Health Organization. Mental health of older adults, 2017. WHO, Geneva, December 2017, pp. 1–6. Available at www.who.int/en/news-room/fact-sheets/detail/mental-health-of-older-adults.

9. Kharicha K, Iliffe S, Harari D, et al. Health risk appraisal in older people 1: Are older people living alone an 'at risk' group? *British Journal of General Practice* 2007; **57**(537):271–6.

10. Roe B, Howell F, Riniotis K, et al. Older people and falls: Health status, quality of life, lifestyle, care networks, prevention and views on service use following a recent fall. *Journal of Clinical Nursing* 2009; **18**(16):2261–72.

11. Sok SR, Yun EK. A comparison of physical health status, self-esteem, family support and health-promoting behaviours between aged living alone and living with family in Korea. *Journal of Clinical Nursing* 2011; **20**(11–12):1606–12.

12. Ng TP, Jin A, Feng L, et al. Mortality of older persons living alone: Singapore Longitudinal Ageing Studies. *BMC Geriatrics* 2015; **15**:126–9. Available at http://dx.doi.org/10.1186/s12877-015-0128-7.

13. Manthorpe J. Caring at a distance: Learning and practice issues. *Social Work and Education* 2001; **20**(5):593–602.

14. National Alliance for Caregiving. Caregiving in the U.S. Washington, DC, 2004. Available at www.caregiving.org/research/caregivingusa/.

15. Cagle JG, Munn JC. Long-distance caregiving: A systematic review of the literature. *Journal of Gerontological Social Work* 2012; **55**(8):682–707.

16. Dickens AP, Richards SH, Greaves CJ, Campbell JL. Interventions targeting social isolation in older people: A systematic review. *BMC Public Health* 2011; **11**:1–22.

17. Ilgaz A, Gozum S. Health promotion interventions for older people living alone: A systematic review. *Perspectives in Public Health* 2019; **10**(11):1–9.

18. Moher D, Liberati A, Tetzlaff J, et al. Preferred reporting items for systematic reviews and meta-analyses: The PRISMA statement. *PLoS Medicine* 2009; **6**(7):e1000097.

19. Passos J, Fonte A, Dias CC, Fernandes L. The needs of older people with mental health problems in a Portuguese psychiatric setting. *International Psychogeriatrics* 2017; **29**(5):845–53.

20. Greaves S, Bhat M, Regan C, et al. The unmet needs of referrals to old age psychiatry liaison services. *Psychogeriatria Polska* 2006; **3**(4):175–82.

21. Miranda-Castillo C, Woods B, Orrell M. People with dementia living alone: What are their needs and what kind of support are they receiving? *International Psychogeriatrics* 2010; **22**(4):607–17.

22. van der Roest HG, Meiland FJM, Comijs HC, et al. What do community-dwelling people with dementia need? A survey of those who are known to care and welfare services. *International Psychogeriatrics* 2009; **21**(5):949–65.

23. Hermsen LAH, Hoogendijk EO, van der Wouden JC, et al. Self-perceived care needs in older adults with joint pain and comorbidity. *Aging Clinical and Experimental Research* 2017; **30**:449–55.

24. Stein J, Liegert P, Dorow M, et al. Unmet health care needs in old age and their association with depression: Results of a population-representative survey. *Journal of Affective Disorders* 2019; **245**:998–1006.

25. Meaney AM, Croke M, Kirby M. Needs assessment in dementia. *Geriatric Psychology* 2005; **20**(4):322–9.

26. Sun X, Lucas H, Meng Q. Associations between living arrangements and health-related quality of life of urban elderly people: A study from China. *Quality of Life Research* 2011; **20**:359–69.

27. Lin LHY. The health status and needs of community elderly living alone. *Journal of Nursing Research* 2002; **10**(3):227–36.

28. Henning-smith C. Quality of life and psychological distress among older adults: The role of living arrangements. *Journal of Applied Gerontology* 2017; **35**(1):39–61.

29. Courtin E, Knapp M. Social isolation, loneliness and health in old age: A scoping review. *Health & Social Care in the Community* 2017; **25**(3):799–812.

30. Mui A, Burnette D. A comparative profile of frail elderly persons living alone and those living with others. *Journal of Gerontological Social Work* 1994; **21**(3–4):5–26.

31. Watari K, Wetherell JL, Gatz M, et al. Long distance caregivers: Characteristics, service needs, and use of a long distance caregiver program. *Clinical Gerontologist* 2006; **29**(4):61–77.

Chapter 6

Needs Assessment of People with Dementia and Impact of Caregiver Burden

Myonghwa Park, Thi-Thanh-Tinh Giap, Miri Jeong, Younghye Go and Dong Young Lee

6.1 Introduction

Population structures are changing in many developed countries, and Korean society is currently one of the fastest ageing worldwide.[1] This circumstance is due to a rapidly decreasing birth rate and an increasing life expectancy in recent decades, and this situation is likely to continue for a prolonged period. A national epidemiological investigation predicted that South Korea will move from an ageing society to a 'superaged' society in only 25 years, from 2000 to 2025, with 46.5% (18.3 million) of the population expected to be older than 65 years by 2067.[1] This demographic change gives rise to substantial challenges in dealing with increased demands on medical services relating to chronic and degenerative diseases, particularly related to the increasing prevalence of dementia in elderly patients (which was 9.2% in 2014).[2] The care needs of community-residing people with dementia are complex and depend on the severity of dementia symptoms, such as cognitive impairment, functional dependencies and behavioural and psychological symptoms.[3]

An 'unmet' need refers to a significant problem requiring intervention or assessment, for which currently no assistance or the wrong kind of help is provided.[4] Because of various limitations related to impairments of cognitive function, failing memory, lack of company, lack of information and psychological distress,[5] people with dementia have multiple unmet needs related to physical, psychological, social and economic issues.[6] Therefore, generating an appropriate instrument to measure both the met and unmet needs of people with dementia is both essential and valuable for health providers and researchers in formulating essential strategies to address the existing common needs. Such an instrument will also be helpful for investigating and evaluating the effects of any interventions

applied. Accordingly, the Camberwell Assessment of Need for the Elderly (CANE),[7] which was adapted from the Camberwell Assessment of Need,[8] has been designed for comprehensive assessments of the environmental, physical, psychological and social needs of the elderly. Translated versions of the CANE have been used successfully in many countries around the world, including Australia,[9] Brazil,[10] Germany,[11] Iran,[12] Poland,[13] Portugal,[14] Netherlands,[15] Spain,[16] and South Korea.[17,18]

The caregiving demands of people with dementia living in their own homes increase as their dementia progresses, including a need for constant protection and observation. Additionally, most family caregivers do not have professional caregiver skills and expertise. Thus, dementia has a negative impact not only on people with dementia but also on their family caregivers, which may lead to a significant burden on the family in the caregiver role.[19] Numerous studies have found that the family caregivers of people with dementia often experience burden related to health and psychological problems, family and social support, information, religious and spiritual needs and practical support needs.[20] South Korea has also been struggling to address this situation of increasing burden and stress in family caregivers of people with dementia.[21,22] Hughes et al.[23] indicated that unmet needs are positively related to caregiver burden; that is, the increasing unmet needs of people with dementia and of family caregivers will lead to increases in caregiver burden. Therefore, meeting the needs of people with dementia could reduce the caregiver burden.[24]

This study was conducted with two purposes: (1) using the Korean version of the CANE (CANE-K) to determine both the met and unmet needs of Koreans with dementia and (2) measuring the burden of family caregivers of people with dementia.

6.2 Methods

6.2.1 Design

This study was based on a cross-sectional survey conducted in Seoul, South Korea.

6.2.2 Participants

The participants were dyads of people with dementia and their primary family caregivers at home. The study randomly selected 656 people with dementia who were registered in the online database of the Seoul Dementia Management Project[25] from June to August 2014 and invited them to participate in the research. All questionnaires were administered via face-to-face interviews conducted by trained research assistants. The survey addressed treatment, caregiving burden and cost issues related to dementia care in community settings. Forty of the 360 dyads of community-residing people with dementia and their families were excluded from the final analysis because 23 were non-family caregivers and 17 had at least 5% of variables with missing data.

6.2.3 Measures

6.2.3.1 Unmet Needs

The CANE-K was used in this study.[17] The CANE consists of 24 items, with each item rated as follows: no need, met need, or unmet need. The CANE assesses the informal and formal help that the older adult receives and the satisfaction with that help. The number of unmet needs was the total number of areas scored as an unmet need. Reynolds et al.[7] found that Cronbach's α for this instrument was 0.87, whereas it was 0.84 in the present study, which used the tool to assess the needs of people with dementia from the perspective of their family caregivers.

6.2.3.2 Caregiving Burden

The Zarit Burden Interview (ZBI) was developed in 1980,[26] and its Korean version (ZBI-K), as translated in 2006,[27] was used to measure personal burden and role burden in this study. Each item ranges from 0 (never) to 4 (nearly always). Cronbach's α for the ZBI-K was previously found to be 0.92,[27] and it was 0.94 overall in this study.

6.3 Results

6.3.1 Demographics

As presented in Table 6.1, the people with dementia were aged 80.0 ± 7.5 years (mean ± standard deviation [SD]), and most of them were female (63.8%). The mean duration of dementia was 3.7 years, and most of the people were diagnosed with Alzheimer's disease (60.8%). Along with dementia, almost all the people had at least one additional disease (91.6%), with a mean number of diseases of 3.1.

The family caregivers were aged 63.7 ± 12.5 years and comprised twice as many females than males. Nearly half of them were spouses of the care recipients (42.0%), followed by daughters (25.4%). The caregivers were spending a mean of 8.5 hours per day caring for people with dementia and had done this for a mean of 3.4 years. Most of the family caregivers (84.3%) lived with the care recipients. More than half of the main caregivers (54.8%) did not have anyone else who helped them look after the care recipient. In terms of perceived health status, only 22% of the caregivers thought they were in good health, and most of them (52.2%) considered that they had a high burden of care costs.

6.3.2 The Needs of People with Dementia

The needs of people with dementia and the source of help are presented in Table 6.2. The number of needs of people with dementia ranged from 0 to 22 out of a total of 24 aspects surveyed, with the following distribution: 1 (0.3%) had no need, 301 (94.1%) had 6 or more needs, 172 (53.8%) had 12 or more needs, and 2 (0.6%) had 22 needs. The number of met needs ranged from 0 to 16, with 311 care recipients (97.2%) having 12 or fewer, 167 (52.2%) having 6 or fewer, and 2 (0.6%) having no need met. The care recipients had an average of 5.09 ± 4.22 unmet needs, with this ranging between 0 and 19: of these, 43 (13.4%) had no unmet needs and 129 (40.3%) had 6 or more unmet needs.

6.3.2.1 Types of Needs

Among the 24 items assessed, the prevalence of no need ranged from 10.3% (memory) to 95.9% (abuse/neglect). Five items had rates of no need of higher than 80%: abuse/neglect (95.9%), alcohol (95.6%), deliberate self-harm (93.4%), accommodation (86.9%) and behaviour (81.6%). Thirteen items had rates of no

Table 6.1 Characteristics of the People with Dementia and Their Family Caregivers

Characteristic	Value
People with Dementia (*n* = 320)	
Age, years	80.0 ± 7.5
≤64	8 (2.5%)
65–74	69 (21.6%)
75–84	147 (45.9%)
≥84	96 (30.0%)
Sex (female)	204 (63.8%)
Duration of dementia, years	3.7 ± 2.0
≤3	234 (73.1%)
4–6	77 (24.1%)
≥7	9 (2.8%)
Number of diseases	3.1 ± 1.6
Type of dementia	
Alzheimer's disease	172 (60.8%)
Other	111 (39.2%)
Family Caregivers (*n* = 320)	
Age, years	63.7 ± 12.5
≤44	21 (6.7%)
45–64	144 (45.7%)
65–74	71 (22.5%)
≥75	79 (25.1%)
Sex (female)	215 (67.2%)
Relationship to patient	
Spouse	134 (42.0%)
Daughter	81 (25.4%)
Son	48 (15.0%)
Daughter-in-law	45 (14.1%)
Other	11 (3.4%)
Duration of caregiving, years	3.4 ± 2.6
≤3	187 (61.7%)
≥4	116 (38.3%)
Duration of caregiving per day, hours	8.5 ± 4.6
≤8	161 (57.3%)
≥9	120 (42.7%)
Co-residence	
Yes	268 (84.3%)
No	50 (15.7%)
Secondary caregiver	
Yes	142 (45.2%)
No	172 (54.8%)

Table 6.1 (cont.)

Characteristic	Value
Perceived health status	
Good	69 (22.0%)
Fair	126 (40.3%)
Poor	118 (37.7%)
Burden of care costs	
High	167 (52.2%)
Moderate	91 (28.4%)
Low	62 (19.4%)

Note: Data are *n* (%) or mean ± SD values.

need of less than 50%: memory, money/budgeting, looking after the home, food, physical health, mobility/falls, daytime activities, company, self-care, continence and eyesight/hearing/communication (in ascending order).

The rate of unmet needs among the 24 items assessed ranged widely, from 0.9% for abuse/neglect to 53.4% for memory. The five items with the highest rates of unmet need were memory (53.4%), money/budgeting (49.4%), daytime activities (46.3%), company (40.3%) and benefit (32.5%). The five items with the lowest rates of unmet need were abuse/neglect (0.9%), alcohol (2.2%), deliberate self-harm (4.1%), accommodation (4.4%) and behaviour (7.5%).

Calculating the percentage of unmet needs relative to the total needs (excluding care recipients with no need) revealed that 7 of the 24 items had percentages higher than 50%: benefit (68.0%), deliberate self-harm (65.0%), daytime activities (62.5%), memory (59.8%), company (58.4%), money/budgeting (58.1%) and intimate relationships (51.6%). The item with the smallest rate was physical health (12.2%), followed by abuse/neglect (27.3%), food (29.2%) and psychological distress (29.8%).

The needs of the family caregivers for psychological distress and information were relatively high, at 64.4% and 38.6%, respectively, whereas the corresponding rates of unmet needs were 25.0% and 11.3%.

6.3.2.2 Sources of Help

Most people with dementia received no or very little help from their family and friends for needs regarding accommodation (78.6%), abuse/neglect (72.7%), information (66.2%) and caring for someone else and benefit (60.5%). Four needs for which they often received help from their family and friends were food,

Table 6.2 Needs of People with Dementia and the Source of Help They Received (n = 320)

Need	No Need	Met Need	Unmet Need	Unmet Need/Total Needs, %	Receiving Help from			Need for Community Services (often/always)
					Family and Friends (no/sometimes)	Services (no/sometimes)	Satisfied	
Accommodation	278 (86.9)	28 (8.8)	14 (4.4)	33.3	33 (78.6)	37 (90.2)	9 (21.4)	18 (43.9)
Looking after the home	59 (18.4)	182 (56.9)	79 (24.7)	30.3	51 (20.4)	188 (75.5)	153 (62.7)	95 (38.9)
Food	65 (20.3)	165 (51.6)	89 (27.8)	29.2	45 (18.4)	178 (73.3)	158 (66.4)	96 (40.3)
Self-care	133 (41.6)	126 (39.4)	60 (18.8)	32.3	33 (18.4)	121 (67.6)	115 (64.6)	78 (44.3)
Caring for someone else	241 (75.3)	48 (15.0)	29 (9.1)	37.2	46 (60.5)	60 (78.9)	33 (43.4)	36 (47.4)
Daytime activities	83 (25.9)	89 (27.8)	148 (46.3)	62.5	101 (44.5)	177 (78.7)	102 (46.5)	114 (51.8)
Memory	33 (10.3)	115 (35.9)	171 (53.4)	59.8	102 (36.6)	213 (76.6)	138 (50.7)	136 (49.8)
Eyesight/hearing/communication	151 (47.2)	97 (30.3)	72 (22.5)	42.6	59 (36.9)	133 (83.1)	83 (52.9)	70 (44.0)
Mobility/falls	82 (25.6)	142 (44.4)	95 (29.7)	40.1	71 (32.0)	171 (77.7)	114 (53.3)	92 (42.8)
Continence	136 (42.5)	90 (28.1)	90 (28.1)	50.0	62 (36.5)	124 (73.4)	94 (56.0)	73 (43.2)
Physical health	65 (20.3)	224 (70.0)	31 (9.7)	12.2	111 (45.3)	202 (82.8)	150 (61.5)	82 (34.2)
Drugs	186 (58.1)	84 (26.3)	47 (14.7)	35.9	30 (23.6)	105 (82.7)	79 (62.7)	43 (34.1)
Psychotic symptoms	194 (60.6)	64 (20.0)	62 (19.4)	49.2	51 (42.1)	93 (76.9)	58 (47.9)	56 (46.7)
Psychological distress	188 (58.8)	92 (28.8)	39 (12.2)	29.8	55 (43.0)	103 (80.5)	53 (42.1)	58 (46.0)
Information	167 (52.2)	102 (31.9)	51 (15.9)	33.3	96 (66.2)	126 (86.9)	84 (58.3)	51 (35.4)
Deliberate self-harm	299 (93.4)	7 (2.2)	13 (4.1)	65.0	8 (42.1)	16 (84.2)	7 (36.8)	6 (31.6)
Inadvertent self-harm	220 (68.8)	50 (15.6)	49 (15.3)	49.5	44 (45.4)	79 (80.6)	45 (45.9)	43 (44.3)
Abuse/neglect	307 (95.9)	8 (2.5)	3 (0.9)	27.3	8 (72.7)	9 (81.8)	1 (9.1)	4 (36.4)
Behaviour	261 (81.6)	35 (10.9)	24 (7.5)	40.7	27 (47.4)	44 (77.2)	17 (29.8)	26 (45.6)
Alcohol	306 (95.6)	7 (2.2)	7 (2.2)	50.0	7 (53.8)	7 (53.8)	6 (46.2)	6 (46.2)
Company	97 (30.3)	92 (28.8)	129 (40.3)	58.4	115 (53.7)	185 (86.4)	90 (43.1)	103 (48.8)
Intimate relationships	191 (59.7)	61 (19.1)	65 (20.3)	51.6	65 (53.3)	106 (86.9)	46 (39.3)	63 (43.3)
Money/budgeting	47 (14.7)	114 (35.6)	158 (49.4)	58.1	58 (22.7)	215 (84.6)	165 (66.8)	85 (34.3)
Benefit	167 (52.2)	49 (15.3)	104 (32.5)	68.0	89 (60.5)	127 (86.4)	37 (11.6)	81 (55.8)
Caregiver's need for information	196 (61.4)	87 (27.3)	36 (11.3)	31.6	85 (73.3)	100 (87.0)	37 (32.7)	53 (46.1)
Caregiver's psychological distress	114 (35.6)	126 (39.4)	80 (25.0)	38.8	144 (73.5)	172 (88.7)	49 (26.1)	97 (50.8)

Notes: Number of unmet needs per person with dementia: 5.09 ± 4.22, range = 0–19. Data are n (%) values except where indicated otherwise.

self-care, looking after the home and money/budgeting (all ≥77.3%).

Most of the care recipients (67.6%) did not receive help or received very little help from services for all of the 24 needs assessed; this particularly included accommodation (90.2%), information and intimate relationships (89.6%) and company and benefit (86.4%).

The rates of family caregivers who received no or very little help from their family and friends were high for needs of both information and psychological distress (about 73.0%). This rate was also high (about 87.0%) for receiving help from services.

6.3.2.3 Satisfaction

Satisfaction rates of care recipients with the help they received (both from family and friends and from services) were relatively low, ranging from 9.1% to 66.8%. The highest rates of care recipients satisfied with the help they received were for money/budgeting (66.8%), food (66.4%), self-care (64.6%), looking after the home (62.7%) and physical health (61.5%). Three needs that almost all care recipients were not satisfied with were abuse/neglect (9.1%), benefit (11.6%) and accommodation (21.4%). Only 26.1% of the caregivers were satisfied with the help they received for their psychological distress, whereas 32.7% were satisfied with this for their information needs.

6.3.2.4 Need for Help from Community Services

Relatively high proportions of care recipients (31.6%–55.8%) thought that help from community services was often or always necessary for their needs. The highest proportions were for benefit (55.8%), daytime activities (51.8%), memory (49.8%) and company (48.8%). Additionally, about half of caregivers indicated that help from community services was often or always necessary.

6.3.3 Burden on Family Caregivers of People with Dementia

As presented in Table 6.3, the overall burden across the 22 items was 1.94 ± 0.92 for each item. The following four items had scores of less than 1.5: 'Does your relative currently affect your relationship with other family members?' (1.24 points); 'Do you feel uncertain about what to do about your relative?' (1.44 points); 'Do you wish you could just leave the care of your relative to someone else?' (1.47 points); and 'Do you feel strained when you are around your relative?' (1.49 points). The following four items had

the highest scores: 'Are you afraid that your relative is dependent upon you?' (3.00 points); 'Do you feel that your relative seems to expect you to take care of him/her as if you were the only one he/she could depend on?' (2.74 points); 'Are you afraid about what the future holds for your relative?' (2.49 points); and 'Do you feel that you will be unable to take care of your relative for much longer?' (2.37 points).

The overall burden score was 42.78 ± 20.30, with a range from 0 to 88. This overall score corresponds to a moderate to severe burden level. Most of the 320 family caregivers of people with dementia who participated in this study were assessed as having a moderate to severe burden (35.3%), followed by those with a mild to moderate burden (30.6%), a severe burden (19.7%) and little or no burden (14.4%).

6.3.3.1 Relationship Between Caregiver Burden and Needs of the Care Recipients

Figure 6.1 presents the items that had highest rates of unmet needs according to burden level. Four items appeared in all four burden groups, with three of these items having rates of unmet needs that increase monotonically from a level of little or no burden through to a severe burden: memory (17.39%, 51.02%, 55.75% and 79.37%, respectively), money/budgeting (21.74%, 40.82%, 57.52% and 68.25%, respectively) and daytime activities (28.26%, 44.90%, 50.44% and 57.14%, respectively). The rate of unmet needs of the remaining item (company) increased from a level of little or no burden (17.39%) to a mild to moderate burden (46.94%), then decreased slightly to a moderate to severe burden (37.17%) and reached the highest rate for severe burden (52.38%).

As presented in Figure 6.2, an increasing number of unmet needs was associated with an increase in level of caregiver's burden. In general, the burden increased gradually from the group with a smaller number of unmet needs to the group with a larger number of unmet needs.

6.4 Discussion

This study identified the needs of people with dementia and their family caregivers, as well as the burden placed on their family caregivers, in a relatively large number of participants (320 dyads). The overall number of unmet needs of the people with dementia in this study was 5.09 ± 4.22, which is higher than those found in several previous studies. In particular, a study conducted in the Netherlands

Table 6.3 Burden on Family Caregivers of People with Dementia (*n* = 320)

ID	Item	Burden Score
1	Do you feel that your relative asks for more help than he/she needs?	1.50 ± 1.28
2	Do you feel that because of the time you spend with your relative you don't have enough time for yourself?	2.28 ± 1.42
3	Do you feel stressed between caring for your relative and trying to meet other responsibilities for your family or work?	2.30 ± 1.27
4	Do you feel embarrassed over your relative's behaviour?	1.88 ± 1.24
5	Do you feel angry when you are around your relative?	1.51 ± 1.21
6	Do you feel that your relative currently affects your relationship with other family members or friends in a negative way?	1.24 ± 1.29
7	Are you afraid what the future holds for your relative?	2.49 ± 1.29
8	Do you feel that your relative is dependent on you?	3.00 ± 1.17
9	Do you feel strained when you are around your relative?	1.49 ± 1.33
10	Do you feel that your health has suffered because of your involvement with your relative?	1.54 ± 1.40
11	Do you feel that you don't have as much privacy as you would like because of your relative?	2.15 ± 1.40
12	Do you feel that your social life has suffered because you are caring for your relative?	2.01 ± 1.38
13	Do you feel uncomfortable about having friends over because of your relative?	1.53 ± 1.50
14	Do you feel that your relative seems to expect you to take care of him/her as if you were the only one he/she could depend on?	2.74 ± 1.40
15	Do you feel that you don't have enough money to care for your relative in addition to the rest of your expenses?	2.06 ± 1.40
16	Do you feel that you will be unable to take care of your relative much longer?	2.37 ± 1.37
17	Do you feel that you have lost control of your life since your relative's illness?	1.53 ± 1.35
18	Do you wish that you could leave the care of your relative to someone else?	1.47 ± 1.34
19	Do you feel uncertain about what to do about your relative?	1.44 ± 1.23
20	Do you feel that you should be doing more for your relative?	2.08 ± 1.28
21	Do you feel that you could do a better job in caring for your relative?	2.08 ± 1.30
22	Overall, how burdened do you feel in caring for your relative?	2.13 ± 1.23
	Average score across the 22 items	1.94 ± 0.92
	Overall score	42.78 ± 20.30, range = 0–88
	Level of Burden	
	Little or no burden (0–20 points)	46 (14.4%)
	Mild to moderate burden (21–40 points)	98 (30.6%)
	Moderate to severe burden (41–60 points)	113 (35.3%)
	Severe burden (61–88 points)	63 (19.7%)

Note: Data are *n* (%) or mean ± SD values.

found that the average numbers of unmet needs were 0.5 and 1.7 for people living in the community, as reported by the people with dementia and their informal caregivers, respectively.[28] In contrast, other studies found that the average numbers of unmet needs in the United Kingdom were 1.17, 2.14 and 2.64 for people living at home, as reported by people with dementia, caregivers and professionals, respectively,[5] and 4.4 for people living in residential care, as reported by trained researchers.[29] These discrepancies may be related to differences in service provision between countries. Korean people with dementia still need to receive appropriate help from both their caregivers and health services when attempting to effectively respond to their existing unmet needs.

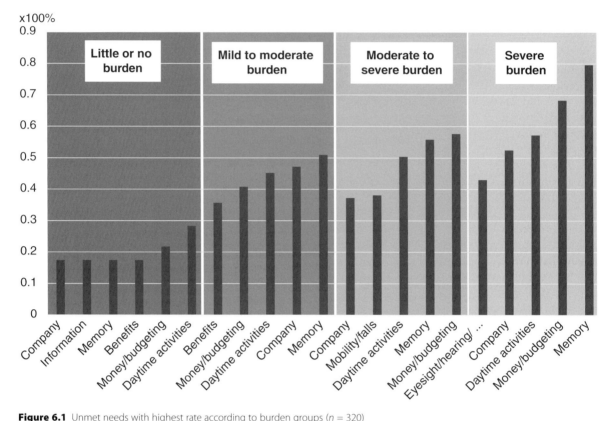

Figure 6.1 Unmet needs with highest rate according to burden groups ($n = 320$)

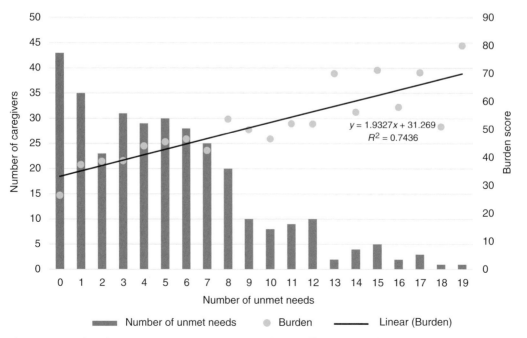

Figure 6.2 Number of unmet needs and burden score according to different groups of number of unmet needs ($n = 320$)

Among the 24 items assessed in this study, the most frequent unmet needs were memory (53.4%), money/budgeting (49.4%), daytime activities (46.3%), company (40.3%) and benefit (32.5%). Three of these five unmet needs were also found to be the most common in previous studies: daytime activities,[5,28-30] company[5,28-30] and memory.[28,29] In contrast, while the rates of unmet needs for money/budgeting and benefit were high in this study, at nearly half and one-third of the participants, respectively, the corresponding rates were very low in both the Netherlands[28] and the United Kingdom.[5,29,30] The most common unmet needs found in other studies of psychological distress,[5,28-30] eyesight/hearing/communication[5,29,30] and information,[5,28] did not exhibit high rates in this study. These variations between the different studies show that different communities have specific problems that need to be addressed. Therefore, besides the needs of people with dementia that appeared at relative high rates, such as physical health (70.0%), looking after the home (56.9%), food (51.6%) and mobility/falls (44.4%), stakeholders should identify appropriate interventions and strategies to respond to the unmet needs as identified in this study.

Regarding the sources of help, family and friends play a primary and important role in meeting the needs of care recipients, the most frequently related to autonomy. However, our findings also indicate a major challenge for further studies and policymakers when the satisfaction of people with dementia for help or assistance received is rated at less than 50% for more than half their needs (i.e., 13 of 24).

In agreement with numerous studies from both South Korea[6,21,31] and other countries,[20,32] this study also indicated that the overall level of burden on family caregivers of people with dementia was mild to moderate and especially that 19.7% participants were evaluated as experiencing severe burden. This is because dementia is a chronic disease that requires long-term care to cope with the complex demands of affected individuals, which leads to a significant burden for the family in the caregiver role. Along with the identified issues that most caregivers were concerned about (Table 6.3), a relationship between the caregiver burden and unmet needs of care recipients was detected. Several needs remained unmet in all four groups of burden levels and gradually increased from little or no burden through to severe burden, including memory, money/budgeting, daytime activities and company. Additionally, the findings demonstrated that an increasing number of unmet needs were associated with an increasing burden score ($R^2 = 0.744$).

The findings of this study are valuable for both researchers and policymakers in the context of the increasing number of people with dementia in South Korea. In particular, the data obtained by this study provides a comprehensive picture of the needs of people with dementia, including indicating the issues that have and have not been well responded to. This information can be used by researchers and policymakers to identify priority strategies to cope with existing needs. These strategies should especially focus on the factors associated with the remaining high rate of unmet needs, such as memory, food, alcohol and company.

Reducing the burden on family caregivers is also an important goal. This would not only help to increase the quality of life of the caregivers but also improve the quality of care for people with dementia. This will help to delay the time to nursing home placement of people with dementia; in other words, it is meaningful for reducing the financial burden for society.[33] The findings of this study indicate that decreasing the number of unmet needs of people with dementia will lead to reducing the burden of their caregivers. This means that efforts aimed at helping to meet the needs of people with dementia will also bring benefits in reducing caregiver burden. As presented in this study, several needs that had large effects on increasing caregiver burden were memory, money/budgeting, daytime activities and company, so further research should emphasise these factors as a priority.

In addressing the limitations of this study, we should mention the differences in the needs reported between people with dementia and other stakeholders, such as caregivers and professionals.[5,28] Therefore, to better reflect the need priorities, future studies should attempt to simultaneously assess the needs based on the personal views of these different groups.

6.5 Conclusion

The people with dementia included in this study had multiple needs, nearly one-fifth of which were not being met, most frequently for memory, money/budgeting, daytime activities, company and benefit. Moreover, a larger number of unmet needs of people with dementia will increase the burden on family caregivers, especially regarding needs related to memory, money/budgeting, daytime activities and company.

Acknowledgements

This study was supported by grants from the Seoul Metropolitan Center for Dementia (Grant 2014–12) and the National Research Foundation of Korea (Grant NRF-2017R1A2B1011044).

References

1. Statistics Korea. The Future Population Projection 2017–2067. Available at www.kostat.go.kr/ portal/korea/kor_nw/1/1/index.board?bmode= read&aSeq=373873 (accessed 30 December 2019).

2. Kim YJ, Han JW, So YS, et al. Prevalence and trends of dementia in Korea: A systematic review and meta-analysis. *Journal of Korean Medical Science* 2014; **29**(7):903–12.

3. Rabins PV, Lyketsos CG, Steele CD. *Practical Dementia Care*. New York: Oxford University Press; 2006.

4. Orrell M, Hancock G. *CANE: Camberwell Assessment of Need for the Elderly*. London: Gaskell; 2003.

5. Miranda-Castillo C, Woods B, Orrell M. The needs of people with dementia living at home from user, caregiver and professional perspectives: A cross-sectional survey. *BMC Health Services Research* 2013; **13**(1):13–43.

6. Park M, Sung M, Kim SK, et al. Multidimensional determinants of family caregiver burden in Alzheimer's disease. *International Psychogeriatrics* 2015; **27**(8):1355–64.

7. Reynolds T, Thornicroft G, Abas M, et al. Camberwell Assessment of Need for the Elderly (CANE): Development, validity and reliability. *British Journal of Psychiatry* 2000; **176**:444–52.

8. Phelan M, Slade M, Thornicroft G, et al. The Camberwell Assessment of Need: The validity and reliability of an instrument to assess the needs of people with severe mental illness. *British Journal of Psychiatry* 1995; **167**(5):589–95.

9. McSweeney K, Jeffreys A, Griffith J, et al. Specialist mental health consultation for depression in Australian aged care residents with dementia: A cluster randomized trial. *International Journal of Geriatric Psychiatry* 2012; **27**(11):1163–71.

10. Sousa RMdM, Scazufca M, Menezes PR, et al. Feasibility and reliability of the elderly version of the Camberwell Assessment of Needs (CANE): Results from the São Paulo Ageing and Health Study. *Brazilian Journal of Psychiatry* 2009; **31**(1):34–8.

11. Stein J, Luppa M, König H-H, Riedel-Heller SG. The German version of the Camberwell Assessment of Need for the Elderly (CANE): Evaluation of content validity and adaptation to the German-speaking context. *International Psychogeriatrics* 2015; **27**(11):1919–26.

12. Salehi R, Davatgaran K, Heidari M, et al. The psychometric properties of the Persian version of the Camberwell Assessment of Needs (CANE) for Iranian elderly people with mental disorders. *Iranian Journal of Ageing* 2018; **13**(2):168–81.

13. Rymaszewska J, Kłak R, Synak A. Camberwell Assessment of Need for the Elderly (CANE): Study of Polish version of the tool. *Psychogeriatria Polska* 2008; **5**(2):105–13.

14. Balsinha C, Marques MJ, Gonçalves-Pereira M. A brief assessment unravels unmet needs of older people in primary care: A mixed-methods evaluation of the SPICE tool in Portugal. *Primary Health Care Research & Development* 2018; **19**(6):637–43.

15. van der Roest HG, Meiland FJ, van Hout HP, et al. Validity and reliability of the Dutch version of the Camberwell Assessment of Need for the Elderly in community-dwelling people with dementia. *International Psychogeriatrics* 2008; **20**(6):1273–90.

16. Mateos R, Ybarzábal M, Garcia M, et al. The Spanish CANE: Validation study and utility in epidemiological surveys. In Orrell M, Hancock G (eds.), *CANE: Camberwell Assessment of Need for the Elderly*. London: Gaskell; 2004:21–8.

17. Park M, Kim SK, Jeong M, et al. Psychometric validation of the Korean version of the Camberwell Assessment of Need for the Elderly in individuals with dementia. *Asian Nursing Research* 2018; **12**(2):106–12.

18. Park M, Choi S, Lee SJ, et al. The roles of unmet needs and formal support in the caregiving satisfaction and caregiving burden of family caregivers for persons with dementia. *International Psychogeriatrics* 2018; **30**(4):557–67.

19. Bakker C, de Vugt ME, van Vliet D, et al. The relationship between unmet care needs in young-onset dementia and the course of neuropsychiatric symptoms: A two-year follow-up study. *International Psychogeriatrics* 2014; **26**(12):1991–2000.

20. Etters L, Goodall D, Harrison BE. Caregiver burden among dementia patient caregivers: A review of the literature. *Journal of the American Academy of Nurse Practitioners* 2008; **20**(8):423–8.

21. Kim M-D, Hong S-C, Lee C-I, et al. Caregiver burden among caregivers of Koreans with dementia. *Gerontology* 2009; **55**(1):106–13.

22. Yong F, McCallion P. Hwabyung as caregiving stress among Korean-American caregivers of a relative with dementia. *Journal of Gerontological Social Work* 2004; **42**(2):3–19.

23. Hughes TB, Black BS, Albert M, et al. Correlates of objective and subjective measures of caregiver burden among dementia caregivers: Influence of unmet patient and caregiver dementia-related care needs. *International Psychogeriatrics* 2014; **26**(11):1875–83.

24. Cleary M, Freeman A, Hunt GE, Walter G. Patient and carer perceptions of need and associations with care-giving burden in an integrated adult mental health service. *Social Psychiatry and Psychiatric Epidemiology* 2006; **41**(3):208–14.

25. Lee DY. Seoul dementia management project and Seoul metropolitan center for dementia. *Journal of Korean Geriatric Psychiatry* 2007; **11**(1):8–11.

26. Zarit SH, Reever KE, Bach-Peterson J. Relatives of the impaired elderly: Correlates of feelings of burden. *Gerontologist* 1980; **20**(6):649–55.

27. Bae K, Shin I, Kim S, et al. Care burden of caregivers according to cognitive function of elderly persons. *Journal of the Korean Society of Biological Therapies in Psychiatry* 2006; **12**(1):66–75.

28. van der Roest HG, Meiland FJ, Comijs HC, et al. What do community-dwelling people with dementia need? A survey of those who are known to care and welfare services. *International Psychogeriatrics* 2009; **21**(5):949–65.

29. Hancock GA, Woods B, Challis D, Orrell M. The needs of older people with dementia in residential care. *Journal of the Psychiatry of Late Life and Allied Sciences* 2006; **21**(1):43–9.

30. Miranda-Castillo C, Woods B, Galboda K, et al. Unmet needs, quality of life and support networks of people with dementia living at home. *Health and Quality of Life Outcomes* 2010; **8**(1):1–14.

31. Kim SK, Park M, Lee Y, et al. Influence of personality on depression, burden, and health-related quality of life in family caregivers of persons with dementia. *International Psychogeriatrics* 2017; **29**(2):227–37.

32. Wharton W, Epps F, Kovaleva M, et al. Photojournalism-based intervention reduces caregiver burden and depression in Alzheimer's disease family caregivers. *Journal of Holistic Nursing* 2019; **37**(3):214–24.

33. Colombo F, Llena-Nozal A, Mercier J, Tjadens F. *Help Wanted? Providing and Paying for Long-Term Care* (OECD Health Policy Studies). Paris: OECD Publishing; 2011.

Crisis and Assessment of Need in Dementia
Development of a Home Treatment Package

Juanita Hoe, Ritchard Ledgerd, Sandeep Toot and Martin Orrell

7.1 Introduction

The population is ageing, and dementia is the greatest global challenge for health and social care in the twenty-first century.[1] A recent review estimated that the financial cost of dementia overall to the United Kingdom is £34.7 billion, and this is set to rise sharply over the next two decades to £94.1 billion in 2040.[2] In the United Kingdom, there are currently around 850,000 people living with dementia, and this is expected to almost triple by 2050.[3] While approximately two-thirds of these people with dementia live in the community,[4] one-third are living alone in their own homes[5] and are supported mainly by their families.[6,7] Dementia symptoms can occur alongside other mental health conditions, including depression and anxiety,[8] together with an increased risk of physical health co-morbidities.[1] The progressive nature of dementia is often coupled with other health and social needs, and management is complex.[9] Given the multifaceted nature of dementia, crises can often occur and lead to hospital admissions and care home placements.[10,11] Consequently, people with dementia account for 42% of people over the age of 70 who experienced unplanned admissions to hospital, rising to 48% of people aged over 80 years.[12] However, people with dementia have poorer outcomes when admitted to hospital, including increased confusion, risk of infection, longer bed stays and lower quality of life.[13]

A national priority in the United Kingdom is to find the best ways to help people with dementia to live well at home.[14] Practice and policy guidance emphasise the need for high-quality, cost-effective mental health services for people with dementia and their carers, which include hospital admission avoidance strategies for older people and the need for leadership, sharing good practice, avoiding duplication and improving standards in social care.[15–18] There is particular focus on the delivery of interventions in a person's own home and avoidance of care home placement, which provides benefits such as improved quality of life and cost-saving efficiencies for health and social care systems. With supporting evidence showing that people with dementia want to be involved in the decision-making process, greater involvement of the person with dementia in the planning of their care and support, education and training for family carers are also advocated.[19,20]

7.2 Causes of Crises for People with Dementia and Their Carers

Defining situations or events which cause crises for people with dementia and their caregivers can be difficult as it often depends on the family carer's subjective judgement.[21] According to Parker and Penhale's model[22] for understanding crises, it is during the state of disequilibrium caused by an emotionally hazardous event that the caregiver is likely to find themself in a crisis state where the usual problem-solving and coping strategies are ineffective, and it is during this stage of disequilibrium that a caregiver should be provided with increased and intensive support to enable them to return to a state of homeostasis.[22,23] Crisis situations are highly dynamic, and there are a number of stressors that can contribute to the development of crisis situations; many are interlinked, reflecting the multifaceted nature of the dementia and its impact on various aspects of daily living activities. In addition, a crisis for people with dementia can result from singular or multiple causes.[24,25] The most frequently described causes of crisis include

- Exacerbation or development of behavioural and psychological problems, including verbal and physical aggression, wandering, inability to control emotions, mood disturbances and disorientation to time, place and person[26–28]
- Physical or chronic health conditions warranting medical attention, including falls, immobility, infection and constipation[29,30]

- Delirium, an acute confusional state that can occur with rapid onset, sometimes caused by infection and/or neurological changes in the brain[29,31]
- An inability to manage daily living skills, living alone, poor social networks, limited insight and severity of cognitive impairment, which include the inability to manage household appliances, maintain a secure home environment and identify risk[25,29,32]
- Carer burden, which is the most significant factor contributing to the institutionalisation of a person with dementia, is usually predicated by a crisis situation[27,28,33–35]

Furthermore, being a caregiver impacts on the social, emotional and quality of life for family carers and becomes more challenging as the disease progresses.[36,37] In addition, carers of people with dementia are more likely to experience depressive symptoms, higher levels of stress and lower ratings of wellbeing.[34]

7.3 Management of Crises in Dementia

Managing crisis situations in a person's home environment often has better outcomes than in a hospital environment, particularly for people with dementia.[15,38,39] People with dementia admitted to hospital can become less independent and are more likely to experience increased levels of disorientation, mainly due to the sudden change in environment. These changes can exaggerate behavioural and psychological symptoms and also increase the risk of developing hospital-acquired infections and falls.[26,40] Interventions aimed at avoiding hospitalisation or delaying care home placement, such as managing difficult behaviours and supporting carer burden, can result in improved quality of life for people with dementia and their family carers, greater independence and economic benefits.[28,41,42]

Crisis intervention models have a role in the identification and management of crisis situations. One of the principles in crisis theory is that although two people can experience the same traumatic event, each person may deal with the situation differently, based on (1) the individual's perception of the situation and (2) the individual's ability to utilise their traditional coping skills.[43] It is important to understand how individuals perceive particular situations and how their subjective response may lead to a crisis event developing. Many of the principles included in crisis interventions models intersect with the goals of case management. The use of case management provides support to people at home and is defined as 'any intervention involving interaction between a case manager and patient-caregiver dyads and providing continuity and advocacy over time, support, information about community services, care and disease evolution, financial and legal advice'.[34] The use of dementia case management decreases the risk of institutionalisation, improves quality of care and lowers distress and burden.[44,45] However, there is debate about the selection and robustness of interventions used to support people at times of crisis and whether or when the case management model is effective.[46] More research is needed to evaluate whether case management is an effective model and to define the interventions that form part of this approach.[47,48]

7.4 Home Treatment and Case Management Interventions

Case management and home treatment interventions are available for people with dementia and their caregivers, but their implementation has not been standardised, and the evidence for case management has shown diversity across the interventions provided.[45,46,49] Although the case management interventions offered have taken a variety of different forms, such as the Medicare Alzheimer's Disease Demonstration,[50] disease management programmes[51,52] and care programmes delivered by district nurses,[47] they have similar goals. Case management interventions have been provided by social services care managers and nurses, who develop care plans for people with dementia and their caregivers using a manual which consists of algorithms linking specific care management actions to assessment results.[51] Other elements of case management interventions include home visits and follow-up telephone calls, increased provision for respite, 24-hour availability of a case worker, counselling, education and training for family caregivers and people with dementia (such as with caregiving and coping strategies) and assistance with improving communication between the family caregivers and health and social services.[47,51,53–56] Such interventions have resulted in higher proportions of community assistance and social support being offered, with improvements in the quality of care and caregiving provided, increased quality of life for people with dementia and the caregiver, lower levels of unmet needs, reduced caregiver burden[51,55,56] and, ultimately, lower rates of institutionalisation.[53–56]

National policy guidance advises that community mental health services for older people need to provide 24-hour home-based crisis support and alternatives to inpatient care.[18,57,58] Despite the emphasis on supporting older people with dementia at home to help maintain their independence and quality of life rather than admitting them to hospital, there is a lack of evidence for alternatives to acute psychiatric admissions for older people.[18,59] However, a pilot project in the United States showed that home treatment crisis interventions for people with dementia are effective for reducing behavioural disturbances, carer burden and hospital and care home admissions.[25] As part of the Support at Home Interventions to Enhance Life in Dementia (SHIELD) research programme,[60] we wanted to create a model that included the most promising interventions and components for an effective home treatment package for dementia. This was achieved through systematically reviewing the literature and undertaking mixed-method approaches with professionals, academics, care workers, the voluntary sector, family carers and people with dementia to establish the best evidence for approaches to support people with dementia and their family carers in crisis at home. Our goal was to identify approaches for intensive home support to help manage crises at home and prevent admission to hospital for people with dementia. This chapter focuses on the development of the home treatment package and establishing its applicability and acceptability for practice.

7.5 Preliminary Work Leading to Development of the Home Treatment Package

In the first phase of the study, we conducted a Cochrane review to evaluate the effectiveness of case management approaches to home support for people with dementia.[45] This review showed evidence that case management is beneficial at improving outcomes for people with dementia and their carers in terms of reduced hospital length of stay at 6 and 12 months, reduced behavioural disturbances at 12 and 18 months, reduced carer burden and improved carer wellbeing. Although case management involves higher use of community services, this may be offset by a lower use of acute services and hospitalisations, but the evidence about how this approach affects overall healthcare costs is not clear. An additional systematic review was undertaken of the risk factors leading to hospital admission in dementia, which found that many acute hospital admissions for people with dementia are potentially preventable but that older people's crisis teams tend to focus on prevention and reducing psychiatric admissions.[61] The review identified a low threshold for early treatment in the community and highlighted the need for recognition of the physical health risks in people with dementia and more integrated working between services for older people's mental health, primary care, social care, intermediate care and hospital liaison. We then conducted a further systematic review of crisis-resolution approaches to support people with dementia at home alongside a scoping exercise of home treatment services for older people with mental health needs to establish a typology of such services.[29] The scoping exercise identified three types of home treatment service models with varying definitions of crisis, and the review found a lack of evidence for the efficacy of crisis-resolution home treatment teams.

The second phase involved three focus groups: one with community mental health practitioners, one with family caregivers and one with people with dementia. The aim of the focus groups was to identify factors precipitating crises and to identify interventions that may help manage crises for people with dementia living at home and their family carers.[24] People with dementia and family carer views provided valuable insights into the most important causes and the most useful interventions to help them cope in times of crisis. Whereas people with dementia were concerned about risks and increased vulnerability associated with declining cognition, they favoured informal support from local networks provided by family, friends and neighbours, memory aids and the use of adaptations to help reduce hazards and allow them to remain at home safely. Family carers understood the range of factors precipitating crises, but their main concerns were increased carer burden, poor carer mental health and lack of support from other family members or other services. Conversely, staff members were more concerned about issues with service organisation and coordination leading to crises. Both family carers and staff members valued carer education, care plans and well-coordinated care. A thematic analysis was undertaken of the responses regarding causes of crisis, which were grouped into five domains: behavioural/psychological, physical health, vulnerability, family carer and environment. A similar analysis was undertaken of the responses regarding interventions, which were grouped into four domains: professional healthcare support, home living environment, social home care and family carer. These themes were used to design a questionnaire for an online survey conducted with a network of key stakeholders to identify the primary causes of crises and interventions which are useful for managing or preventing a crisis in dementia.[62] The stakeholders included health, social and emergency care practitioners, academics, people with dementia and family carers and voluntary sector and care workers. Participants ranked the main causes of crisis, interventions that can prevent a crisis and interventions that can be useful in a crisis in order of importance. Although there were differences of opinion across the different stakeholder groups, we found that wandering, falls and infection were highly rated as risk factors for crises across all stakeholder groups. Education and support for family carers and home care staff were highly valued for preventing crises, whereas well-trained home care staff, communication equipment, emergency contacts and access to respite were highly valued for managing crises.

7.6 Development of the Home Treatment Package

Phase three of the study comprised development of the home treatment package for people with dementia and their family caregivers. A modified Delphi process[63,64] was used that involved consensus approaches to develop a home treatment manual with case examples through several iterations (draft version 1, draft version 2, draft version 3 and draft version 4) and field testing to assess the practicality and applicability of its use in practice. Traditionally, the Delphi process involves two iterations of questionnaires and feedback reports. The respondents complete the questionnaires and reports independently, and there is no formal discussion among them.[65] Consensus is reached after the results of the second round of questionnaires, which are modified using the results from the first round. The Delphi process is a good technique for generating a high quantity of ideas, but a shortfall is that there is no opportunity for face-to-face problem solving, and conflicts are not resolved; thus there are advantages in meeting and discussing the findings if necessary and appropriate.[65–68] As a result, for development of the home treatment package, an adapted version of the classic Delphi process was used (see Figure 7.1).

Our process of consultation and consensus was implemented through

1. Initial drafting of the home treatment manual and home treatment package (HTP) advisory protocol with case examples and a training package

2. A consensus conference with key stakeholders to consult on draft version 1 of the home treatment manual and the HTP advisory protocol

3. Case review workshops using case discussions conducted with multidisciplinary expert practitioners to review and develop draft version 2 of the home treatment manual

4. Ratification and consensus activity with practitioners, family carers and experts in the field of home treatment using draft version 3 of the home treatment manual

5. Field testing of the manual in practice using draft version 4 of the home treatment manual

7.7 Development of the Home Treatment Package with Case Examples

An initial manual of home treatment interventions was drafted incorporating the results of the systematic reviews,[29,45,61] scoping visits to home treatment teams,[29] focus groups[24] with community mental health practitioners, people with dementia and family carers and the results of the online survey[62] sent out to the stakeholder network. The contents of the home treatment manual incorporated the different stages of crisis, which consisted of algorithms to ensure coherent application of the interventions. This included the HTP advisory protocol for assessing people with dementia and their family carers at times of crises. The term *advisory protocol* was used because home treatment is shaped by preferences and choice, where in comparison with disease management there is less technological certainty about the necessary courses of action. The HTP advisory protocol focused on assessment of need using the Camberwell Assessment of Need for the Elderly (CANE)[69] and incorporated the Threshold Assessment Grid (TAG) risk assessment[70] and a care planning tool with case examples. From the findings of the online survey,[62] we were able to develop a table of interventions that were incorporated into the home treatment manual (draft version 1) and included the four categories professional healthcare, home living environment, social home care and

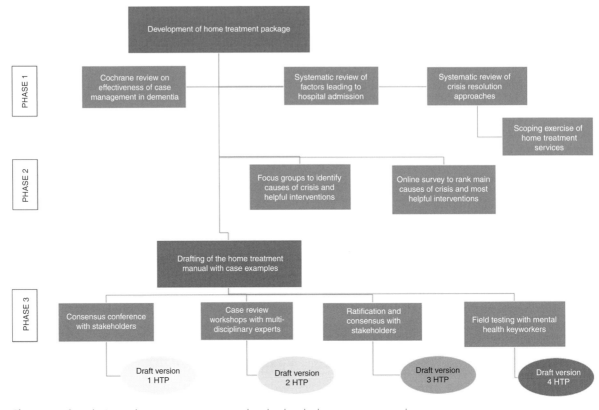

Figure 7.1 Consultation and consensus processes used to develop the home treatment package

family care support. Within the table, the interventions were presented in two distinct formats: a list of interventions which prevent a crisis and a list of interventions considered most useful in a crisis. Alongside the development of the manual, we created a training package for using the HTP advisory protocol and delivering the interventions.

7.8 Consensus Conference

A consensus conference was organised to consult on the home treatment manual (draft version 1) and the HTP advisory protocol. The consensus conference was conducted based on the ideas embedded in the consensus development conference model of bringing together independent academics, people with dementia and family carers, practitioners and experts in the field to obtain general agreement on the efficacy and safety of health technologies.[71] Invitations were sent to 99 people from our database of key stakeholders. Twenty-three participants attended the consensus conference. Of these, there were 15 (65.2%)

practitioners, 3 (13.0%) family carers, 1 (4.3%) voluntary organisation representative, 1 (4.3%) representative from the independent sector and 3 (13.0%) representatives from professional bodies. Additional email consultation was undertaken with a further 13 academics and practitioners on the stakeholder database who were unable to attend. The consensus conference consisted of a series of short presentations on development of the manual, a review of the existing evidence about crisis interventions and the organisation of home treatment teams in South East England. Participants were divided into five small working groups comprising a mix of delegates and facilitated by members of the research team. Each working group was assigned one of the categories, behavioural/psychological, physical health, vulnerability, family carer and environment, and were asked to select the top five interventions for all the factors in each of these categories. Participants selected the top five interventions that were most likely to be useful in a crisis (immediate) and those most likely to prevent a crisis (preventative) from the table of interventions

Table 7.1 Example of Interventions for the Problem Areas Contributing to Crises in Dementia (Behavioural/Psychological Domain)

Behavioural/ Psychological	Most Likely to Be Useful in a Crisis (Immediate)	Most Likely to Prevent a Crisis (Preventative)
Wandering/ purposeful walking	• Family carer education/training (advice, support, coping and relaxation techniques) • Immediate/emergency provision of care (e.g., same day) • Specialist assistive technology (gas sensor, flood/falls/smoke detector, entrance/exit sensor) • Specialist assessments by a member of the multidisciplinary team • Physical health checks	• Specialist assistive technology (gas sensor, flood/falls/smoke detector, entrance/exit sensor) • Engaging in purposeful activities around the home • Prompts/cues/reminders placed in different areas around the home • Flexible provision of services (e.g., home care services extended over 24 hours) • Presence of a family carer
Physical aggression	• Specialist assessments by a member of the multidisciplinary team • Immediate/emergency provision of care (e.g., same day) • Emergency access to respite in the home • Family carer education/training (advice, support, coping and relaxation techniques) • Access to healthcare professionals 24 hours a day	• Family carer education/training (advice, support, coping and relaxation techniques) • Support/specialist training for healthcare practitioners in understanding dementia • Physical health checks • Specialist training for home care staff in how to work with people with memory problems and their family carers
Sleep disturbance/ excessive night-time activity	• Access to healthcare professionals 24 hours a day • Specialist assessments by a member of the multidisciplinary team • Flexible provision of services (e.g., home care services extended over 24 hours) • Emergency access to respite in the home • Emergency access to respite in a residential care home	• Specialist assistive technology (gas sensor, flood/falls/smoke detector, entrance/exit sensor) • Maintaining a routine of daily living tasks • Engaging in purposeful activities around the home • Family carer education/training (advice, support, coping and relaxation techniques)
Verbal aggression	• Specialist assessments by a member of the multidisciplinary team • Immediate/emergency provision of care (e.g., same day) • Emergency access to respite in the home • Family carer education/training • Access to healthcare professionals 24 hours a day	• Family carer education/training (advice, support, coping and relaxation techniques) • Support/specialist training for healthcare practitioners in understanding dementia • Physical health checks • Specialist training for home care staff in how to work with people with memory problems and their family carers

generated through the online stakeholder survey (see Table 7.1). This exercise helped identify how resources should be deployed and used and those which are most helpful in making home treatment approaches effective.

Following selection of the top five interventions, participants discussed a range of 'high risk' case examples and were asked to articulate best practice care packages and responses using draft version 1 of the home treatment manual. The participants applied the HTP advisory protocol to these case vignettes and identified relevant interventions as part of the care planning process. Participants had the choice of selecting interventions from the top five and the fuller table

of interventions identified as being most likely to be useful in a crisis (immediate) and those most likely to prevent a crisis (preventative) or to identify additional interventions if these were thought to be more appropriate. Of the 10 case vignettes that were completed, all the care plans were completed using both immediate or preventive interventions selected from either the top five interventions identified for that factor and the fuller list of interventions. The feedback from the participants was unanimous in that the top five interventions selected were relevant and appropriate for meeting the needs identified in the case vignettes. The responses from consensus conference participants were amalgamated into a glossary of interventions which were incorporated into a further version of the home treatment manual (draft version 2).

7.9 Case Review Workshops

To test the initial suitability and application of using the home treatment manual (draft version 2) and HTP advisory protocol, we held five case review workshops in Manchester, Hertfordshire and East London. Organised workshop days were arranged at each site with expert multidisciplinary team members consisting of consultants, doctors, nurses, occupational therapists, social workers and psychologists, and structured discussions about carefully selected case examples took place. The participants explored how these referrals/admissions could have been better managed or potentially avoided within existing service resources and also identified key areas of unmet needs and the absence of essential resources. The key reasons for admissions were categorised (see Table 7.2), and potential strategies to meet the needs of a person with dementia or family carer were identified. We used the CANE needs assessment tool[69] to identify unmet and met needs and provide a standardised framework for prioritising interventions. This process helped to identify any additional key attributes in crisis occurrences and management that may have been overlooked previously during the development process. Forty-five healthcare practitioners participated in these sessions and applied the HTP advisory protocol to clinical situations and cases they had managed. The workshops generated both

Table 7.2 Categorisation of the CANE Items to the Five Critical Domains that Contribute to Crises

CANE	Behaviour	Physical	Vulnerability	Family Carer	Environment
Accommodation			✓		✓
Looking after the home			✓		✓
Food			✓		✓
Self-care			✓		
Caring for someone else			✓		
Daytime activities	✓		✓	✓	
Memory	✓		✓	✓	✓
Eyesight/hearing/communication		✓			
Mobility/falls		✓	✓		✓
Continence		✓			
Physical health		✓			
Drugs	✓	✓	✓		
Psychotic symptoms	✓				
Psychological distress	✓		✓		
Information				✓	
Deliberate self-harm	✓				
Inadvertent self-harm	✓	✓	✓		✓
Abuse/neglect	✓		✓	✓	
Behaviour	✓				
Alcohol	✓	✓	✓		✓
Company			✓		✓
Intimate relationships	✓				
Money/budgeting			✓		
Benefits			✓		
Carers need for information				✓	
Carers psychological distress				✓	

individual and group feedback on use of the home treatment manual in addition to 40 completed cases using the HTP advisory protocol.

Feedback and suggestions from the case review workshops were used to draft version 3 of the home treatment manual. Participants were generally positive about using the manual but were not always clear about the relationship between the need (CANE)[69] and risk (TAG)[70] assessments and how to interpret the scores and prioritise the unmet needs. It was subsequently agreed that the needs should be prioritised as immediate/high/moderate/low to provide clarity. Participants also had difficulty matching the unmet need to the cause of crisis, so the use of bracketed examples was re-introduced, such as: 'chronic diseases' (e.g., heart conditions, chest problems, diabetes) and 'inability to identify potential risks' (e.g., leaving the front door open, bogus callers). There was some sensitivity around wording, such as use of the term *wandering* and the phrase *family carer is abusing the person with dementia/memory problems*, and the term *abusing* was replaced with *neglecting*. The care plan within the HTP advisory protocol was thought to lack adequate detail, and this was renamed as a care planning tool to distinguish its primary purpose of informing the care planning process. Navigating through the printed manual was difficult for those unfamiliar with its design and structure, and the introduction of tabs or colour coding was suggested, which we adopted for the glossary in the revised manual.

7.10 Ratification and Consensus on the Home Treatment Manual

Consultation to validate and ratify the home treatment manual (draft version 3) was undertaken with 50 people from our stakeholder network database of practitioners, family carers and experts in home treatment. All were sent a copy of the manual. Stakeholders were asked to provide comments and feedback to the research team on the format, layout and content of the manual and HTP advisory protocol. In particular, participants were asked to focus attention on sections 1 and 2 of the manual, which described (1) how the advisory protocol was developed and its intended use and (2) the structure and content of the HTP advisory protocol and to provide feedback on the relevance of the contents and their applicability to practice in managing or preventing

crisis situations in dementia. Participants could comment on the whole manual if they preferred and were asked to test the practicality and applicability of using it by applying the HTP advisory protocol to one of the case vignettes in the manual.

The questions asked were:

1. Are you happy with the manual in its current form?
2. Was the manual easy to read and follow?
3. Was there anything you did not you like about the manual?
4. Do you think anything is missing from the manual?
5. Is there anything you would change in the manual?
6. Any other comments?

We received feedback on the home treatment manual from 15 respondents in total; these were 13 practitioners including: mental health nurses, occupational therapists, clinical psychologist, a service manager, consultant psychiatrist, an occupational therapy practice officer and one family carer. About half of those consulted stated that they had read the complete manual, and three respondents read the manual and applied the vignettes. Although there were some concerns about the length of the home treatment manual, there was a general consensus about the manual being informative, easy to read and use, relevant to practice, comprehensive and suitable for use.

> I like the document. It is a time-consuming read as it is detailed and at times complex. … However, it is relevant and supports good practice. – Respondent 13

Several comments were received about the general usefulness of the manual in managing crises in dementia and the structure it offered while still offering individualised care.

> The Manual contains some valid points and offers excellent advice around crisis situations and managing crisis situations. – Respondent 4
>
> I think the manual is useful as it provides a very structured approach without being overly prescriptive, medicalised or complicated. I think it is a very practical manual but still very person centred. – Respondent 11

Participants particularly liked the inclusion of evidence-based interventions to promote and measure effective practice in crisis teams.

I have worked in a crisis team for over two years, and to see the 'process' formalised and based on evidence is excellent. – Respondent 5

This manual will probably help in auditing the effectiveness of crisis teams, something which we found quite difficult. – Respondent 6

Participants were keen to see the manual introduced into practice and could also envisage its applicability in other areas of practice.

I think this is an excellent piece of work and look forward to the next phase. – Respondent 10

What a fantastic piece of work this is. I can really see some benefit in how we could roll some of this out within physical health care services, especially in our Community Inpatient Services, where we see quite a bit of dementia. – Respondent 12

Based on the feedback received, changes were made to the manual, which included reducing its length, changing wording where requested and adding in a quick-access guide and list of abbreviations and acronyms (draft version 4).

7.10.1 Field Testing the Home Treatment Package in Practice

Field testing was conducted to assess the practicality and applicability of using the home treatment manual (draft version 4) and HTP advisory protocol in practice. We wanted to assess whether the home care package could be delivered as intended and tested aspects of feasibility, tolerability and efficacy through applying the HTP advisory protocol to people with dementia experiencing a crisis situation. We recruited 17 mental health practitioners who support people with dementia either approaching or in crisis situations and who would use the HTP advisory protocol with their clinical caseload. The practitioners were recruited from home treatment teams and community mental health teams in the North West of England and North East London. Consent was obtained from the service managers for the clinical area and from the practitioners for their participation in the study. We provided a training day on the use of the manual and HTP advisory protocol, and supervision structures were agreed on before the field testing commenced. Supervision was provided by clinical research staff to the teams through telephone and email contact. The HTP advisory protocol (see Figure 7.2) was implemented on initial assessment following referral to the service or when the risk of hospital admission was identified for people with dementia who were known to the service.

For the 17 practitioners trained to implement the HTP advisory protocol, only 10 practitioners (59%) used the HTP advisory protocol, 3 were based in community mental health teams and 7 in home treatment teams. The reasons for the remaining 7 practitioners not using the HTP advisory protocol were due to change of role/promotion (2), does not care coordinate/admin role (1), declined (1), medium-/long-term sickness (2) and unknown (1).

We collected data from the HTP advisory protocol over an eight-week period, which was applied at two time points: on initial assessment and on evaluation. It was applied to 21 clinical cases of people with dementia and caregiver dyads. The clinical cases were either new referrals to the older person's mental health service or existing cases which had been identified as approaching or experiencing a crisis situation. The data included the following clinical outcomes for the person with dementia: the number of unmet needs, the level of risk determined and the number of admissions to hospital or to care homes. All information was anonymised and used to evaluate the ability of practitioners to use the manual and HTP advisory protocol with clinical cases. Of the 21 HTP advisory protocols collected, 21 of 21 forms were completed with 100% accuracy for the TAG[70], the CANE[69] and the care planning tool, with 16 of 21 forms being completed for the discharge care planning tool.

Feedback was collected from the practitioners about their use of the HTP advisory protocol through completion of the adherence-to-protocol questionnaire and an individually completed questionnaire. Only 2 of 10 practitioners completed the adherence-to-protocol questionnaire, and 8 of 10 practitioners provided feedback using the questionnaire, 2 of whom completed the questionnaire jointly. The reason for the remaining 2 practitioners being unable to provide feedback was absence or leave from work.

Question 1: When asked if the home treatment manual and HTP advisory protocol is suitable for purpose in its current form, one respondent answered that they strongly agreed, four agreed and two disagreed. With two respondents commenting that they found the CANE useful to use, five thought the advisory protocol was time-consuming to use and three encountered coding difficulties.

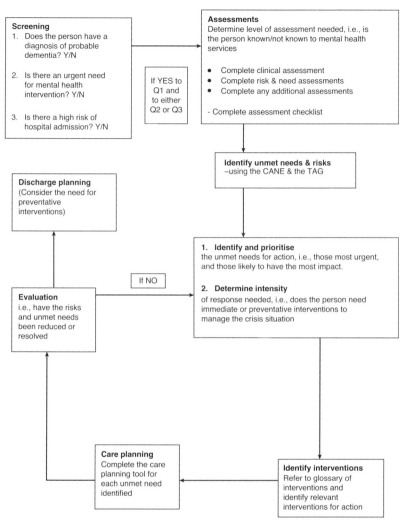

Screening
1. Does the person have a diagnosis of probable dementia? Y/N
2. Is there an urgent need for mental health intervention? Y/N
3. Is there a high risk of hospital admission? Y/N

If YES to Q1 and to either Q2 or Q3

Assessments
Determine level of assessment needed, i.e., is the person known/not known to mental health services

- Complete clinical assessment
- Complete risk & need assessments
- Complete any additional assessments

- Complete assessment checklist

Identify unmet needs & risks
–using the CANE & the TAG

Discharge planning
(Consider the need for preventative interventions)

Evaluation
i.e., have the risks and unmet needs been reduced or resolved

If NO

1. Identify and prioritise
the unmet needs for action, i.e., those most urgent, and those likely to have the most impact.

2. Determine intensity
of response needed, i.e., does the person need immediate or preventative interventions to manage the crisis situation

Care planning
Complete the care planning tool for each unmet need identified

Identify interventions
Refer to glossary of interventions and identify relevant interventions for action

Figure 7.2 Home treatment package advisory protocol pathway

Question 2: When asked if the home treatment manual is easy to read, follow and apply, six respondents agreed and one was unsure, with one respondent commenting on the manual's usefulness.

It is thorough and well thought out. It is good to have a tool to use that is comprehensive and standardised – it reinforces our current practice.

Question 3: When asked if they thought anything is missing from the home treatment manual, five respondents stated no, one did not answer and one stated yes, and this was because

The CANE doesn't cover sleep problems.

A further comment was received from one respondent about the language used in the glossary of interventions:

I found that the terminology relating to the codes was broad enough to encompass all the identified actions on the care plan.

Question 4: When asked if there is anything you would change in the home treatment manual, one respondent stated no, one did not answer and five stated yes. With three respondents stating that the manual is too long, two respondents wanted easier reference systems and two stated that the manual needed a more simplified step-by-step guide to completing the documents. Additional comments were about the usefulness of the manual for less experienced clinicians and the need for familiarity with its application.

I can see the value of the manual and protocol for new or inexperienced staff in order to standardise practice. However, in order for it to be workable, it needs to be used regularly by these practitioners so that it becomes second nature to use.

For those professionals who are inexperienced with working with people with dementia, the manual provides a guide of helpful interventions to consider.

7.11 Discussion

This study demonstrates the usefulness of involving a broad range of stakeholders in the shaping of care planning approaches for dementia. Our initial consultation in the second phase allowed us to create a package of effective home treatment interventions by determining what healthcare practitioners in either mental or physical health services, experts in home treatment, people with dementia and family carers consider to be the key causes of crises in dementia and what interventions they judge as being most helpful in managing or preventing the crisis situations. Our consultation exercises within the consensus conference allowed us to build on the results of the online survey and collectively link the most relevant interventions to specific factors that cause crises in dementia. Immediate interventions are critical in resolving crises in dementia, which are often complicated and multi-factorial situations because of co-morbidity and safety issues.[72] Whereas preventive interventions are important as the degenerative and complex nature of dementia and its impact on families mean that the support and care provided should be sustainable and offer stability in the longer term.[18] Overall there was general agreement about what factors are most likely to result in crises and what is helpful to manage such situations. The involvement of people with dementia and family carers was key to this process, and with interventions being deemed relevant and acceptable, this increases the likelihood of concordance with care plans in crisis situations.

The case review workshops and consensus process enabled the home treatment package to be further improved to prepare it to a level where it was ready for field testing in clinical practice. Although there were concerns about the length and additional work involved, it was regarded as easy to use and practical to apply in clinical situations. However, despite its usefulness, within the field testing, people found completion of the HTP

advisory protocol to be a time-consuming process. This was largely due to it being a novel process, in addition to having to implement the HTP advisory protocol alongside the current care planning procedures. Just over half the practitioners implemented the HTP advisory protocol, and those who were unable provided reasons for not doing so. Reasons included absence from work, change in role and lack of care coordination responsibility. Only one practitioner declined to use the HTP advisory protocol. This suggests that the HTP advisory protocol was acceptable clinically and that the tool may have become less burdensome once the practitioners become more familiar with its structure, and it is the only care pathway in use. Some practitioners were not able to complete the discharge care planning tool and stated that this was because the person with dementia was in their care for longer than the eight weeks, which was the time frame for the field testing. This is significant because the concept for crisis management is short-term intensive intervention,[73] but this is clearly not always possible because of the complexity and interaction between people with dementia and their family carer needs.[46] Nonetheless, including a comprehensive needs assessment tool such as the CANE[69] was found particularly helpful, and the multiperspective rankings for met and unmet needs assisted with readily identifying the most urgent areas for action. Furthermore, it became apparent that when priority areas of unmet needs were dealt with first, it had the consequential impact of successfully resolving issues for less pressing areas of unmet need.

Recommendations were made to shorten the manual and to provide a shorter, more simplified version with a step-by-step flowchart to guide practitioners through the process. Conversely, although it was suggested that some of the detailed descriptions at the beginning of the manual that provided context for the development process were not required, the manual was also acknowledged as being especially beneficial for practitioners inexperienced in working with people with dementia in crisis. Further recommendations were that if the home treatment package were to be implemented in clinical practice, then an electronic or online format would be easier to use. This was deemed a relevant and compelling point as the use of technology has become more prominent within modern National Health Service (NHS) healthcare. The provision of effective and efficient electronic health records (EHRs) is pivotal to enabling the NHS's transformation to digital healthcare provision and has proved its greatest challenge.[74] An electronic version of the home treatment package could help to optimise the 'thought-flow' (clinical decision-making) and the 'workflow' (clinical pathway) required to ensure that EHRs can be used successfully.[74]

7.12 Limitations

A lower number of people than expected participated in the individual consensus and consultation activities and took part in the field testing. This was unfortunate but understandable as the NHS was undergoing significant change and the organisations and staff invited identified difficulties in finding the time to attend. Nevertheless, we consulted with a wide network of stakeholders, and the participants who were involved in the consensus activities offered a useful and meaningful contribution and allowed us to effectively complete the consultation exercises.

7.13 Implications for Practice

Dementia is a complex syndrome that affects all aspects of individuals' and their carers' lives, including impacting on co-morbid conditions and carer burden, which can lead to crisis events.[25] In addition, crises faced by people with dementia and their families are complicated and distressing.[75] Interventions therefore need to be flexible and tailored to both the individual person's needs and the crisis situation.[18,72] Using the HTP advisory protocol can help practitioners by providing a systematic approach to identifying individualised and appropriate interventions that can help resolve the relevant issues contributing to the crisis. Prompt and effective crisis resolution may, in turn, lead to the avoidance of unnecessary or inappropriate hospital admissions and delays in care home placement. Potential benefits are therefore indicated for people with dementia and family carers through wider implementation of the home treatment package within practice.

7.14 Implications for Research

Our study created a model of intensive home support which can be used for managing crisis situations in dementia and offers potential opportunities for future research. We tested the relevance and applicability of using the home treatment package in practice, and the feedback about its usefulness and acceptability was positive, and it provided a useful framework for practitioners. Before the HTP advisory protocol can be introduced into practice, further evaluation of its clinical effectiveness is needed and will be undertaken within a more definitive clinical trial.[76] Future research could also help address the evidence gap for involving people without carers in studies using case management and care planning interventions.[39]

7.15 Conclusion

The use of mixed-method consultation and consensus activities with a wider range of stakeholders was effective in enabling us to successfully develop and revise the home treatment manual and to establish the HTP advisory protocol as a potentially useful tool for clinical practice. The inclusion of people with dementia and family carers was particularly beneficial in identifying interventions in dementia that are relevant and preference based. Furthermore, the ability to produce meaningful and individualised care plans in crisis situations has the potential for improving patient outcomes. Further research is needed, however, to show the effectiveness of applying the HTP advisory protocol within practice.

7.16 SHIELD Home Treatment Manual

Copies of the SHIELD Home Treatment Manual are available from Juanita Hoe (email: juanita.hoe@city.ac.uk).

Acknowledgements

This project was undertaken as part of the National Institute for Health Research (NIHR)–funded Support at Home: Interventions to Enhance Life in Dementia (SHIELD) programme (Grant RP-PG-0606–1083). This report presents independent research commissioned by the NIHR under its Programme Grants for Applied Research scheme (Grant RP-PG-0606–1083). The sponsor of this research programme is the North East London NHS Foundation Trust (NELFT).

References

1. Livingston G, Sommerlad A, Orgeta V, et al. Dementia prevention, intervention, and care. *Lancet* 2017; **390**(10113):2673–734.

2. Wittenberg R, Knapp M, Hu B, et al. The costs of dementia in England. *International Journal of Geriatric Psychiatry* 2019; **34**(7):1095–103.

3. Prince MJ. *World Alzheimer Report 2015: The Global Impact of Dementia: An Analysis of Prevalence, Incidence, Cost and Trends.* London: Alzheimer's Disease International; 2015.

4. Schneider J, Hallam A, Murray J, et al. Formal and informal care for people with dementia: Factors associated with service receipt. *Aging & Mental Health* 2002; **6**(3):255–65.

5. Miranda-Castillo C, Woods B, Galboda K, et al. Unmet needs, quality of life and support networks of people with dementia living at home. *Health and Quality of Life Outcomes* 2010; **8**(1):132–4.

6. Schulz R, Martire LM. Family caregiving of persons with dementia: Prevalence, health effects, and support strategies. *American Journal of Geriatric Psychiatry* 2004; **12**(3):240–9.

7. Dowrick A, Southern A. *Dementia 2014: Opportunity for Change.* London: Alzheimer's Society; 2014. Available at www.alzheimers.org.uk/sites/default/files/migrate/downloads/dementia_2014_opportunity_for_change.pdf.

8. Korczyn AD, Halperin I. Depression and dementia. *Journal of the Neurological Sciences* 2009; **283**(1–2): 139–42.

9. Hutchings R, Carter D, Bennett K. *Dementia – The True Cost: Fixing the Care Crisis.* London: Alzheimer's Society; 2018. Available at www.alzheimers.org.uk/sites/default/files/2018–05/Dementia%20the%20true%20cost%20-%20Alzheimers%20Society%20report.pdf.

10. National Institute for Health and Care Excellence. Transition between inpatient hospital settings and community or care home settings for adults with social care needs. National Institute for Clinical Excellence [online], December 2015. Available at www.nice.org.uk/guidance/ng27.

11. Gallagher D, Ni Mhaolain A, Crosby L, et al. Dependence and caregiver burden in Alzheimer's disease and mild cognitive impairment. *American Journal of Alzheimer's Disease & Other Dementias* 2011; **26**(2):110–14.

12. Sampson EL, Blanchard MR, Jones L, et al. Dementia in the acute hospital: Prospective cohort study of prevalence and mortality. *British Journal of Psychiatry* 2009; **195**(1):61–6.

13. Health Foundation Spotlight on dementia care: Improving care for people with dementia. Health Foundation Improvement Report, London; 2011. Available at www.health.org.uk/publications/spotlight-on-dementia-care.

14. Department of Health. *Prime Minister's Challenge on Dementia 2020: Implementation Plan.* London: Department of Health; 2015. Available at www.gov.uk/government/publications/prime-ministers-challenge-on-dementia-2020.

15. National Audit Office. Improving dementia services in England: An interim report. Stationery Office, London; 2010. Available at www.nao.org.uk/wp-content/uploads/2010/01/091082.pdf.

16. Department of Health. Dementia commissioning pack [online], 2011. Available at http://dementia.dh.gov.uk/dementia-commissioning-pack-launched/.

17. House of Lords Select Committee on Public Service and Demographic Change. Ready for ageing report. Stationery Office, London; 2013. Available at https://publications.parliament.uk/pa/ld201213/ldselect/ldpublic/140/140.pdf.

18. National Health Service. Five-year forward view. London; 2014. available at www.england.nhs.uk/five-year-forward-view/.

19. Dementia Action Alliance. Dementia statements: National dementia declaration. London; 2016. Available at www.dementiaaction.org.uk/nationaldementiadeclaration.

20. Menne HL, Whitlatch CJ. Decision-making involvement of individuals with dementia. *Gerontologist* 2007; **47**(6):810–19.

21. Gräßel E, Adabbo R. Perceived burden of informal caregivers of a chronically ill older family member. *GeroPsych* 2011; **24**(3):143–54.

22. Parker J, Penhale B, *Forgotten People: Positive Approaches to Dementia Care.* Farnham, UK: Ashgate Publishers; 1998.

23. Parker J. Crisis intervention: A practice model for people who have dementia and their carers. *Practice* 2007; **19**(2):115–26.

24. Toot S, Hoe J, Ledgerd R, et al. Causes of crises and appropriate interventions: The views of people with dementia, carers and healthcare professionals. *Aging & Mental Health* 2013; **17**(3):328–35.

25. Johnson DK, Niedens M, Wilson JR, et al. Treatment outcomes of a crisis intervention program for dementia with severe psychiatric complications: The Kansas Bridge Project. *Gerontologist* 2013; **53**(1):102–12.

26. Sörensen S, Duberstein P, Gill D, Pinquart M. Dementia care: Mental health effects, intervention strategies, and clinical implications. *Lancet Neurology* 2006; **5**(11):961–73.

27. George K. Psychiatric admission in dementia care: Cultural and social factors may determine outcome. *Asian Journal of Psychiatry* 2010; **3**(2):73–5.

28. Eska K, Graessel E, Donath C, et al. Predictors of institutionalization of dementia patients in mild and moderate stages: A 4-year prospective analysis. *Dementia and Geriatric Cognitive Disorders Extra* 2013; **3**(1):426–45.

29. Toot S, Devine M, Orrell M. The effectiveness of crisis resolution/home treatment teams for older people with mental health problems: A systematic review and scoping exercise. *International Journal of Geriatric Psychiatry* 2011; **26**(12):1221–30.

30. Vroomen JM, Bosmans JE, van Hout HP, de Rooij SE. Reviewing the definition of crisis in dementia care. *BMC Geriatrics* 2013; **13**(1):1–12.

31. Mukaetova-Ladinska EB, McKeith IG. Delirium and dementia. *Medicine* 2004; **32**(8):44–7.

32. Philp I, McKee KJ, Armstrong GK, et al. Institutionalization risk amongst people with dementia supported by family carers in a Scottish city. *Aging & Mental Health* 1997; **1**(4):339–45.

33. Pinquart M, Sörensen S. Differences between caregivers and noncaregivers in psychological health and physical health: A meta-analysis. *Psychology and Aging* 2003; **18**(2):250–67.

34. Pimouguet C, Lavaud T, Dartigues JF, Helmer C. Dementia case management effectiveness on health care costs and resource utilization: A systematic review of randomized controlled trials. *Journal of Nutrition, Health & Aging* 2010; **14**(8):669–76.

35. Wolfs CA, Kessels A, Severens JL, et al. Predictive factors for the objective burden of informal care in people with dementia: A systematic review. *Alzheimer Disease & Associated Disorders* 2012; **26**(3):197–204.

36. Grau H, Graessel E, Berth H. The subjective burden of informal caregivers of persons with dementia: Extended validation of the German language version of the Burden Scale for Family Caregivers (BSFC). *Aging & Mental Health* 2015; **19**(2):159–68.

37. Sutcliffe CL, Giebel CM, Jolley D, Challis DJ. Experience of burden in carers of people with dementia on the margins of long-term care. *International Journal of Geriatric Psychiatry* 2016; **31**(2):101–8.

38. National Collaborating Centre for Mental Health. Dementia: Supporting people with dementia and their carers in health and social care (Clinical Guideline 42). National Institute for Health and Clinical Excellence, London; 2006. Available at www.nice.org.uk/guidance/cg42.

39. National Institute for Health and Clinical Excellence. Dementia: Assessment, management and support for people living with dementia and their carers (NICE Guideline NG97). National Institute for Health and Clinical Excellence, London; 2018. Available at www.nice.org.uk/guidance/ng97.

40. George J, Long S, Vincent C. How can we keep patients with dementia safe in our acute hospitals? A review of challenges and solutions. *Journal of the Royal Society of Medicine* 2013; **106**(9):355–61.

41. Yaffe K, Fox P, Newcomer R, et al. Patient and caregiver characteristics and nursing home placement in patients with dementia. *Journal of the American Medical Association* 2002; **287**(16):2090–7.

42. Banerjee S, Wittenberg R. Clinical and cost effectiveness of services for early diagnosis and intervention in dementia. *International Journal of Geriatric Psychiatry* 2009; **24**(7):748–54.

43. Roberts AR, ed. *Crisis Intervention Handbook: Assessment, Treatment, and Research.* Oxford, UK: Oxford University Press; 2005.

44. Tam-Tham H, Cepoiu-Martin M, Ronksley PE, et al. Dementia case management and risk of long-term care placement: A systematic review and meta-analysis. *International Journal of Geriatric Psychiatry* 2013; **28**(9):889–902.

45. Reilly S, Miranda-Castillo C, Malouf R, et al. Case management approaches to home support for people with dementia. *Cochrane Database of Systematic Reviews* 2015; **1**(1):1–150.

46. Clarkson P, Hughes J, Roe B, et al. Systematic review – Effective home support in dementia care, components and impacts, stage 2: Effectiveness of home support interventions. *Journal of Advanced Nursing* 2018; **74**(3):507–27.

47. Koch T, Iliffe S, Manthorpe J, et al. The potential of case management for people with dementia: A commentary. *International Journal of Geriatric Psychiatry* 2012; **27**(12):1305–14.

48. Jansen AP, van Hout HP, Nijpels G, et al. Effectiveness of case management among older adults with early symptoms of dementia and their primary informal caregivers: A randomized clinical trial. *International Journal of Nursing Studies* 2011; **48**(8):933–43.

49. Backhouse A, Richards DA, McCabe R, et al. Stakeholders perspectives on the key components of community-based interventions coordinating care in dementia: A qualitative systematic review. *BMC Health Services Research* 2017; **17**(1):1–11.

50. Miller R, Newcomer R, Fox P. Effects of the Medicare Alzheimer's Disease Demonstration on nursing home entry. *Health Services Research* 1999; **34**(3):691–714.

51. Vickrey BG, Mittman BS, Connor KI, et al. The effect of a disease management intervention on quality and outcomes of dementia care: A randomized, controlled trial. *Annals of Internal Medicine* 2006; **145**(10):713–26.

52. Chien WT, Lee YM. A disease management program for families of persons in Hong Kong with dementia. *Psychiatric Services* 2008; **59**(4):433–6.

53. Eloniemi-Sulkava U, Notkola IL, Hentinen M, et al. Effects of supporting community-living demented patients and their caregivers: A randomized trial. *Journal of the American Geriatrics Society* 2001; **49**(10):1282–7.

54. Gaugler JE, Kane RL, Kane RA, Newcomer R. Early community-based service utilization and its effects on institutionalization in dementia caregiving. *Gerontologist* 2005; **45**(2):177–85.

55. Chu P, Edwards J, Levin R, Thomson J. The use of clinical case management for early stage Alzheimer' patients and their families. *American Journal of Alzheimer's Disease & Other Dementias* 2000; **15** (5):284–90.

56. Challis D, von Abendorff R, Brown P, et al. Care management, dementia care and specialist mental health services: An evaluation. *International Journal of Geriatric Psychiatry* 2002; **17**(4):315–25.

57 Department of Health, Care Services Improvement Partnership. Everybody's business – Integrated mental health services for older adults: A service development guide. London; 2005. Available at www.scie-socialcareonline.org.uk/everybodys-business-integrated-mental-health-services-for-older-adults-a-service-development-guide/r/a11G00000017vMyIAI.

58. Royal College of Psychiatrists. Raising the standard – Specialist services for older people with mental illness: Report of the faculty of old age psychiatry. Royal College of Psychiatrists, London; 2006.

59. Draper B, Low LF. What is the effectiveness of acute hospital treatment of older people with mental disorders? *International Psychogeriatrics* 2005; **17**(4):539–55.

60. Orrell M, Hoe J, Charlesworth G, et al. Support at Home – Interventions to Enhance Life in Dementia (SHIELD): Evidence, development and evaluation of complex interventions. *Programme Grants for Applied Research* 2017; **5**(5):1–84.

61. Toot S, Devine M, Akporobaro A, Orrell M. Causes of hospital admission for people with dementia: A systematic review and meta-analysis. *Journal of the American Medical Directors Association* 2013; **14**(7):463–70.

62. Ledgerd R, Hoe J, Hoare Z, et al. Identifying the causes, prevention and management of crises in dementia: An online survey of stakeholders. *International Journal of Geriatric Psychiatry* 2016; **31**(6):638–47.

63. Fink A, Kosecoff J, Chassin M, Brook RH. Consensus methods: Characteristics and guidelines for use. *American Journal of Public Health* 1984; **74**(9):979–83.

64. Murphy MK, Black NA, Lamping DL, et al. Consensus development methods, and their use in clinical guideline development. *Health Technology Assessment (Winchester, England)* 1998; **2**(3):i–88.

65. Ven AH, Delbecq AL. The effectiveness of nominal, Delphi, and interacting group decision making processes. *Academy of Management Journal* 1974; **17**(4):605–21.

66. Jones J, Hunter D. Qualitative research: Consensus methods for medical and health services research. *British Medical Journal* 1995; **311**(7001):376–80.

67. Hoffmann TC, Glasziou PP, Boutron I, et al. Better reporting of interventions: Template for intervention description and replication (TIDieR) checklist and guide. *British Medical Journal* 2014; **348**(g1687):1–12.

68. Dalkey N, Helmer O. An experiential study of group opinion prepared for United States Air Force Project Rand. Santa Monica; 1963.

69. Reynolds T, Thornicroft G, Abas M, et al. Camberwell Assessment of Need for the Elderly (CANE): Development, validity and reliability. *British Journal of Psychiatry* 2000; **176**(5):444–52.

70. Slade M, Powell R, Rosen A, Strathdee G. Threshold Assessment Grid (TAG): The development of a valid and brief scale to assess the severity of mental illness. *Social Psychiatry & Psychiatric Epidemiology* 2000; **35**(2):78–85.

71. Perry S, Kalberer Jr JT. The NIH consensus-development program and the assessment of health-care technologies: The first two years. *New England Journal of Medicine* 1980; **303**(3):169–72.

72. Parker J, Bradley, G. *Transforming Social Work Practice in Assessment, Planning Intervention and Review.* Exeter, UK: Learning Matters; 2003.

73. Knox K, Roberts A. The crisis intervention model. In Coady N, Lehmann P (eds.), *Theoretical Perspectives for Direct Social Work Practice: A Generalist-Eclectic Approach*, 3rd ed. New York: Springer; 2007:183–202.

74. Imison C, Castle-Clarke S, Watson R, Edwards N. *Delivering the Benefits of Digital Health Care.* London: Nuffield Trust; 2016. Available at www.atmedics.com/wp-content/uploads/2016/02/nuffield-trust-delivering-the-benefits-of-digital-care-17-02-2016.pdf.

75. Michon A. Crisis intervention in dementia. *Psychologie & NeuroPsychiatrie du vieillissement* 2006; **4**(2):121–5.

76. Stanyon M, Streater A, Coleston-Shields D, et al. Protocol for the development of an evidence-based 'best practice model' for teams managing crisis in dementia. *Journal of Medical Internet Research Research Protocols*; 2019. Available at https://preprints.jmir.org/preprint/14781.

8

Needs of People with Young-Onset Dementia

Christian Bakker and Britt Appelhof

Key Points

- In young-onset dementia, a family-oriented approach during the caregiving trajectory will increase the likelihood that a fit between care needs of all family members and help and support can be achieved.
- Although the use of standardised instruments for the assessment of needs of people living with young-onset dementia is not common in clinical practice, a pilot study shows that the systematic assessment of specific needs and types of support available was perceived as very valuable by both people with young-onset dementia and their paid and family caregivers.
- With some alterations, the Camberwell Assessment of Need for the Elderly (CANE) appears a complete and thorough instrument that can also be used for the assessment of needs in people with young-onset dementia.

8.1 Introduction

In the past decade, there has been a growing interest among policymakers, researchers and clinicians in individuals living with dementia at a young age. However, no consensus currently exists about what age should actually be considered young.[1] In recent literature addressing the specific issues that younger people living with dementia encounter, often the age of 65 is used as the cut-off age to distinguish younger individuals from those living with dementia at an older age. That said, the age of 65 is a rather arbitrary choice and is largely based on people retiring from work around this particular age in most Western countries. One could argue that age by itself does not distinguish adults who develop dementia early in life from those who develop dementia in old age. Also, aspects such as vitality, social engagement, work and other life-phase-specific aspects determine how dementia affects people's lives. With dementia occurring earlier in life, the impact of the dementia will also be different and, with that, will also result in different needs in the person with dementia as well as other family members. When asked, people living with young-onset dementia also consider themselves distinct from those developing dementia at old age[2] and consider their needs to be different as well.

Mainstream dementia services are not well equipped to address the specific needs of people with young-onset dementia and their family members.[3] This is mainly due to the fact that these services have been developed with the needs of frail older people with dementia in mind. However, although the numbers of people living with dementia at a young age are relatively low compared to dementia in old age, the limited number of available prevalence studies do suggest that this is not a group that can be ignored. An Australian study showed an overall prevalence of 68.2 per 100,000 population in the 30- to 64-year age group.[4] This study also showed that with advancing age, the risk also increases exponentially with 11.6 cases per 100,000 for the 30- to 44-year age group to 132.9 cases per 100,000 for the 45- to 64-year age group. These findings are similar to those of a recent study done in Norway, with estimates of 76.3 cases per 100,000 at risk in the 30- to 64-year age group and 163.1 cases per 100,000 in the 45- to 64-year age group.[5] In the Norwegian study, Alzheimer's disease was found to be the most common cause of dementia in younger individuals, with 56% of all people in this study having Alzheimer's dementia. This means that a larger proportion of people with young-onset dementia have dementia due to another cause. There is a large variation in causes of dementia at a younger age with an equally large variation in presentation, for instance, causes with predominantly behavioural changes such as in the behavioural variant of frontotemporal dementia and very uncommon causes with a progressive course such as metabolic disorders in younger individuals. This stresses the need to explore the specific needs of younger individuals and their families who live with dementia from a broader perspective and perhaps also evaluate current instruments used to inventory needs for the use in people with young-onset dementia.

8.2 Needs of Younger People Living with Dementia

In young-onset dementia there is a substantial delay in the time to diagnosis, which, among other things, has been related to the relatively low prevalence and the many different causes of dementia in younger people.[6] In a large Dutch longitudinal study, the Needs in Young-Onset Dementia (NeedYD) study, exploring the course of dementia in 217 people with young-onset dementia, the time from first symptoms to diagnosis was found to be 4.4 years compared to 2.8 years in individuals with late-onset dementia.[7] A more recent study in Australia, the Improving Service Provision for Younger Onset Dementia (INSPIRED) study, found similar results with a mean time to diagnosis of 4.7 years.[8] In young-onset dementia, neuropsychiatric symptoms instead of cognitive symptoms are often key symptoms in the first stages of the disease, which is rather different from late-onset dementia.[9] As a result, symptoms are often not recognised as symptoms of possible dementia.

Symptoms are often misinterpreted as depression, burnout or job-related strain or even marital difficulties. As a result, people with young-onset dementia are often referred to a psychologist or psychiatric service,[10] and although it is very likely that there will also be symptoms related to stress or depression present, people might not be able to benefit from psychological treatment. Generally, when symptoms eventually worsen or people encounter healthcare professionals who suspect that the symptoms could be a sign of dementia, they are referred to an appropriate diagnostic service. Fortunately, in the past decade, awareness about dementia at a young age has increased in many countries and with that also the likelihood that earlier recognition of dementia symptoms in the young will improve, hopefully shortening the time to diagnosis.

A timely diagnosis is essential because it allows people to start grieving and process how the disease will affect their life. Moreover, people will only initiate healthcare services once they experience their needs as related to dementia, and a match between these needs and existing healthcare services is possible. Because of the delay in the diagnostic trajectory, the process of reflecting on how to live well with dementia and preparing for what lies ahead is delayed as well, while at the same time problems and the accompanying burden will often already be significant. This proves to be a challenge for healthcare professionals involved in young-onset dementia because at the time of diagnosis people are often not yet ready to initiate healthcare services, but a further delay in the initiation of such services is unwanted. This might explain in part why younger people with dementia underuse formal care services[11] and why in young-onset dementia the larger extent of all care is provided by the primary caregiver.[12]

How people with dementia perceive their needs very much relates to people's perception of their own lives, how they were used to living before the onset of dementia and the way the dementia affects the different domains of life, such as daytime activities or social life. In a younger life phase, most people, among other things, will have a job, a mortgage or other long-term financial obligations; will be bringing up children and will have an active social life. People will also still think about the future and how they will spend their lives in this future. This affects how people think about their own needs once a diagnosis of dementia has been established. In people with young-onset dementia, there is a marked loss of a sense of self and identity.[13] This is one of the key issues influencing the way people perceive their needs. For instance, most people at the time of first symptoms or diagnosis will still have a job. However, most people unfortunately lose their job around this time as well, creating a loss of the ability to interact with colleagues, feel useful and have something to do. In most cases, people will perceive that there is no meaningful alternative available, resulting in unmet needs in several domains of their life. Furthermore, people with young-onset dementia often experience difficulties in obtaining the appropriate benefits or even find themselves not eligible for receiving these welfare benefits.[14] This results in financial and legal difficulties, which underlines the importance of professional support aimed at providing appropriate information about legislation, procedures and possible benefits, as well as practical support.

With advancing age, people generally learn how to cope with the loss of certain abilities and how to depend on others. Even in normal ageing this is not always easy. We know from research on subjective needs that people with dementia express needs in domains of life that refer to their general well-being, for instance, regarding how to deal with the fact that they have dementia and less often to domains that refer to instrumental needs.[15] In young-onset dementia there is a sudden role change from being a financial provider, parent, friend or caregiver for elderly parents to someone who depends on the care of others. This causes distress, often resulting in depressive symptoms, resistance to care or conflicts with other family members. When asked, people with young-onset dementia experience high levels of psychological distress. In the NeedYD study we mentioned earlier, one-third of all participants mentioned that they experienced psychological distress, and approximately 12% of these individuals felt that no appropriate support was available for them to reduce this distress.[16] Caregivers in this study reported even higher levels of psychological distress in their relative. This underlines the importance of support groups and psychological support for young people living with dementia. However, it also stresses the importance of initiatives such as DemenTalent and the Spankracht project (Bielderman et al., personal communication, 2020), aimed at supporting people with dementia by showing how to feel useful again and focus on the positive aspects in life and their abilities that still exist.[17]

In the NeedYD study, 40% of participants with young-onset dementia also mentioned the need for information about their dementia and the care options that were available to them. More than half of them expressed that, in their opinion, they had not yet received appropriate information. In comparison with all other domains that were assessed, they expressed the largest proportion of unmet needs in this particular area. Caregivers in this study rated the need for information in their relative as unmet less often. This difference might very well be related to the fact that people with dementia do not always remember the information that has been provided. However, from our clinical experience with support groups for younger people with dementia, we know that people feel that healthcare professionals and caregivers often have difficulty in tailoring information to their needs. Moreover, the way this information is delivered does not always comply with how information can most easily be processed by someone with dementia. Furthermore, people with young-onset dementia often express in support groups that they feel that information is kept from them and that they are not involved in care decisions as much as they would like to be. Whereas it might be the intention of caregivers or healthcare professionals to shield the person with dementia from issues that might trouble them, people with young-onset dementia often find it difficult when they are not involved in care decisions or when information is kept from them. In young-onset dementia, the proportion of people with more intact disease awareness is likely to be higher compared to late-onset dementia.[18] This suggests that we have to establish how to involve younger individuals more closely in advance care planning, how to tailor information to their particular needs and how to deliver this information to them.

Participants in the NeedYD study also often indicated unmet needs in the domain of intimate relationships, for instance, having someone to talk to as well as their sexual needs. People with young-onset dementia often find it difficult to discuss this subject with other people, particularly their own spouse or other people close to them. They often feel embarrassed to raise the subject or experience feelings of guilt towards their spouse, who they believe is already burdened enough. By contrast, whereas the person with dementia might want to engage in sexual activity, their spouse might not feel comfortable engaging in sexual activity because of issues such as incontinence or may feel unsure whether or not these activities are still with mutual consent. Also, spouses often find it difficult to address these themes in a discussion, even though they feel that intimacy and changes in the sexual relationship affect the quality of the spousal relationship. Children often feel uncomfortable in bringing up the subject of intimacy and sexuality with their parent or are not aware that any need in this particular area might be present. This suggests that healthcare professionals should try to support overcoming any taboos that might be there by addressing this issue at some point during the caregiving trajectory.

The NeedYD study also showed that approximately 80% of all participants experienced needs in the domain of mobility and that 16% felt that needs in this area remained unmet. Unmet needs in this particular area were most often related to difficulties in the ability to travel independently. Being able to drive or use other means of transportation is very important for people with dementia, but particularly so in younger individuals. This relates to both autonomy and the ability to sustain a social life and hobbies. Furthermore, it often proves difficult to arrange support in this area, for instance, the support of a volunteer or affordable taxi service. At the same time, in many cases people with young-onset dementia will not accept help in this area because they want to retain their independence and autonomy for as long as possible.

8.3 The Needs of Family Members of People with Young-Onset Dementia

In young-onset dementia, a family-oriented approach aimed at supporting the family in how to live well with dementia is needed. The primary caregiver is often the spouse, and in many cases, children will also be closely involved during the caregiving process. In the period prior to diagnosis, these families experience many difficulties, for instance, in dealing with behavioural changes in their relative, financial problems and a diagnostic trajectory that is a long and winding road. In retrospect, when asked about the period prior to diagnosis, caregivers often feel that they have been neglected by healthcare professionals.[7,19] This can prove to be an important barrier later on during the caregiving trajectory to seek help from healthcare professionals. Once a diagnosis has been established, there is often a lack of fit between the needs of the family and services on offer. Mainstream dementia services will have a focus on the person with dementia and, to some extent, the primary caregiver. However, it is unlikely that these services will have a focus on other family members related to the person with dementia, such as children, brothers and sisters or parents. Also, in these services, a focus on the difficulties that are directly related to a younger life phase is often lacking. A family-oriented approach in services on offer and in advance care planning will increase the likelihood that a fit between care needs of all family members and help and support can be achieved during the caregiving trajectory.

8.4 The Needs of Spousal Caregivers

Although a diagnosis of dementia can cause a lot of grief in caregivers, the diagnosis is often also perceived as an explanation for the difficulties they have experienced in the period prior to diagnosis.[10] After a diagnosis has been established, caregivers express a need for information about what to expect in the period that lies ahead, about the course of the dementia and about care options that are available to them.[20] Caregivers also indicate that a lack of disease awareness in the person with dementia poses an important barrier for informal care and the initiation of professional healthcare services, such as home or day care. This is especially true for frontotemporal dementia, one of the most common subtypes in young-onset dementia. However, impaired disease awareness will also occur in other subtypes of dementia during the course of the disease, even at an early stage of the disease. However, clinical experience shows that in many individuals with young-onset dementia, disease awareness and awareness of the daily consequences of the dementia are relatively intact for a longer period of time. This especially appears to apply to individuals with Alzheimer's disease, in whom disease awareness remains intact for a longer period of time during the course of the dementia compared to individuals with dementia at an old age.[18] This allows caregivers to involve their relative more closely during the caregiving process and also discuss care options with them. At the same time, caregivers often have difficulty in dealing with the grief caused by awareness in their loved one. Healthcare professionals should be aware that caregivers often experience a dilemma regarding whether or not to involve the person with dementia or shield them from things that are going on and care decisions that have to be made. However, involvement of the person with dementia in care decisions will enhance their sense of control over their own situation and also support them in their acceptance of formal care.

The majority of all care in people with young-onset dementia is provided by spouses.[12] Children are sometimes also involved, but only in relatively few cases will they act as the primary caregiver. A recent study into the underuse of formal care services in people with young-onset dementia found that despite the fact that in nearly every case services were offered to the caregivers, two-thirds of study participants chose not to use any of these services.[21] Also, in this study, no association was found between demographic or participant characteristics and service use. However, qualitative analyses showed that a lack of perceived need, lack of availability and young-onset-specific barriers (including ineligibility, unaffordability, lack of security and lack of childcare) were commonly reported as reasons for not using these services. Despite the fact that caregivers of people with young-onset dementia report that they have family, friends and neighbours, they also indicate that in many cases these people are not involved in any of the care activities.[12] Caregivers also express that other people are also often unaware of or inattentive to the difficult circumstances of the caregiver and the burden caused by caring for someone with dementia while at the same time performing other duties, for instance, related to work, running a household or caring for children or parents. This causes many caregivers to experience feelings of loneliness and to be reluctant to ask others to help. Healthcare professionals should therefore aim at supporting caregivers with information on how to inform others nearby about the caregiving situation and how to involve them at some point during the caregiving trajectory to offer themselves some respite from the caregiving situation.

As said earlier, caregivers are faced with the difficult task of combining informal care with other roles and responsibilities related to work, parenting or caring for children or parents. This adds to the burden already experienced by the loss of a future perspective and the loss of reciprocity within the spousal relationship. Caregivers find themselves having to adapt to a role change from being a partner to, as they often express this themselves, a fulltime nurse. The ability of caregivers to accept this role change and adapt to the caregiving situation influences their perception of the care needs of their relative as well as their own needs.[22] Spousal caregivers often experience difficulties in how to regain a life of their own. Because they are involved in caregiving tasks all day and are constantly occupied by problems at hand, there is little room to think of their own needs and desires. Besides the need for support in how to adapt to the caregiving role, spousal caregivers also have a strong need to share experiences with others in a similar situation. For instance, many caregivers experience difficulties around whether or not to engage in a new relationship with another partner, how to involve children in caregiving tasks and whether or not to allow themselves to take time off from caring. Attending support groups with other caregivers who understand what it means to care for someone with young-onset dementia can help. The advice of peers is sometimes more effective than the advice of healthcare professionals, especially support of peers regarding transitions in care, such as

initiating home care or day care and the decisions that are involved with these transitions is essential. This likely also allows for a timelier initiation of care services.

The delay in the initiation of formal care services in people with young-onset dementia applies to institutionalisation in particular. The time to institutionalisation in people with young-onset dementia is nearly nine years from disease onset, which is doubled compared to the time to institutionalisation for older individuals.[23] Institutionalisation is often postponed by caregivers until their relative has advanced dementia. Many caregivers feel that dementia services and nursing homes in particular are not well equipped to provide appropriate care for their relative and are also hesitant about institutionalising their relative because of the stigma attached to such services. This might also be related to the fact that these young caregivers are more likely to believe that they are able to cope and provide care at home for an extended period of time because they themselves are still young. Another explanation might be that in many cases the person with dementia will not be inclined to agree with institutionalisation. At the same time, many caregivers experience feelings of guilt that they cannot continue to care for their loved one at home. These feelings might also be reinforced by reactions of family members, friends or other people who feel that the caregiver chooses to institutionalise their relative too soon.

8.5 Needs of Children and Other Family Members

One of the key issues in people with young-onset dementia relates to the fact that in many cases children, brothers and sisters of the person with dementia and even parents also are involved. Children are often young adults and teenagers, and for a small proportion of cases, they might still be very young. Especially when children are still living at home, they will very much be aware of all the issues at hand. We know from a recent study exploring the needs of children of a parent with young-onset dementia that children's experience of having a parent with dementia affects their lives to a large extent.[24] Children in this study experienced that there were many changes in the relationships between family members, negatively influencing their wellbeing. It also proved difficult for them to be involved in care duties and combining these duties with other responsibilities in their lives, such as going to school or work. We know that children are often very concerned about their healthy parent but also often avoid discussing the dementia and any issues at hand because they do not want to burden their parent.[25] However, communicating within the family about the dementia, care decisions and whether or not each family member feels able to deal with the changes that are caused by the dementia and care duties might enhance their ability to manage and deal with the dementia as a family. The study by Millenaar et al.[24] also showed that children often postpone their own plans, for instance, delaying their study plans or moving out. This is concerning because such decisions might influence their own future much more than they might realise. Children in this study often used avoidant coping strategies while at the same time expressing that they were in need of support themselves. Next to the need for support in how to adapt to the caregiving situation, children indicated that reliable information about the dementia was lacking and that they needed practical support in how to deal with behavioural problems or other changes in their parent.[24] They also indicated that communication and social support were key elements to them, but these were often lacking. Children also have to deal with uncertainty about whether or not they themselves are at risk for developing dementia at a younger age. This adds to the burden children already experience because they gradually lose their parent to dementia and are not able to somehow reverse this.[26] Specific support for children of people with young-onset dementia is largely lacking in most countries. This underlines the importance of the development of specific support for children, such as peer support groups or support in finding the appropriate information. We know from the study by Millenaar et al.[24] that children might be reluctant to use support from healthcare professionals. E-health programmes such as those currently being developed in the Netherlands specifically for children of a parent with young-onset dementia (www.caregiverbalance.eu/home/en/) might prove to be an important step forward in the support of children. The intervention consists of a combination of an online course and support from a healthcare professional already involved with the family. Although Caregiver Balance was originally developed as an intervention for spouses, it is currently tailored and evaluated for the support of children of younger people living with dementia.

Next to children, other family members are also involved in young-onset dementia, such as parents, brothers and sisters and other relatives. Unfortunately, little is known about the needs of these family members as this remains a highly under-researched area. Knowledge about the specific needs and wants of these family members is essential for the development of appropriate support. Currently, there is an ongoing study regarding the aforementioned Caregiver Balance project aimed at the development of a specific intervention for this particular group.[24a] This study shows that topics that should be addressed in the support of other family members include how to deal with grief, management of behavioural and cognitive changes in the person with dementia, communication and genetics.

8.6 Use of the CANE in Young-Onset Dementia

The use of standardised instruments for the assessment of needs of people living with young-onset dementia such as the CANE is not common practice, not in research nor in clinical practice. This might be related to the fact that these instruments have been developed with a different population in mind, and clinicians or researchers might be hesitant to use these instruments in young-onset dementia. Recently, in the Behaviour and Evolution of Young-Onset Dementia Part 2 (BEYOND II) study, a multicomponent care programme was developed aimed to improve the management of behavioural problems such as agitation, apathy and depression in institutionalised people with young-onset dementia.[27] Because of the strong association between unmet needs and the occurrence and persistence of behavioural problems people with in young-onset dementia,[16] adding a specific instrument for the detection of unmet needs to the care programme was believed to be an important prerequisite for the analysis of possible causes of the behaviour. Because the CANE is a widely used instrument, it was decided to incorporate this instrument in the care programme. Because little was known about the use of the CANE with this particular population, a pilot study was performed.

Most institutionalised people with young-onset dementia have advanced dementia. Even when sufficient communicative abilities are present, interviewing people with more advanced dementia would likely reduce the validity of self-reported results. As a result, use of the CANE as an observational tool was explored during the pilot. As a first step in preparation of the pilot, a panel group discussion was organised with both researchers and healthcare professionals with specific expertise on young-onset dementia. Healthcare professionals included a psychologist, a case manager, a social worker and a registered nurse. The panel discussion was held to investigate whether the 24 domains included in the original CANE were also relevant for institutionalised people with young-onset dementia and whether or not additional domains should be included.

Participants in the panel group discussion indicated that the needs of institutionalised people with young-onset dementia occur in the same domains as in older people, and no additional domains were felt necessary. However, participants suggested that adaptations to the existing domains were needed. The domain memory was perceived as incomplete, especially because in young-onset dementia a focus on memory might not be unproblematic because, for instance, in frontotemporal dementia, which is highly prevalent in younger individuals, memory issues might not be the most prominent symptom. Besides memory, other cognitive abilities could also be impaired, such as planning, attention, theory of mind and visual-spatial skills, which could result in unmet needs. Therefore, it was suggested to replace memory with cognitive impairment. Furthermore, because the instrument would be used in institutionalised people with young-onset dementia, participants suggested removing the domains medication and alcohol. They felt that medication prescriptions and alcohol use are closely monitored in residents, reducing the risk for unmet needs in these particular areas. Participants also indicated that all costs of care are covered for institutionalised people with dementia in the Netherlands, and additional benefits are redundant. Therefore, no unmet needs in the domain welfare benefits were expected. Furthermore, participants suggested that psychotic symptoms and psychological distress could be combined in one domain called *mental health*. Also, they suggested combining the areas safety by accidental self-harm and safety by abuse/neglect in one area called *safety*. Participants also suggested that behavioural problems should not be included in the instrument when incorporating the instrument in the care programme for the treatment of behavioural problems because behavioural problems are considered a cause or effect of unmet needs in the care programme.

Besides the aforementioned, suggestions were also made by participants for the examples in the original CANE used to recognise needs and identify types of support to meet unmet needs. Participants felt that some examples were not applicable to the nursing home setting and needed to be adapted. For instance, in the domain accommodation, being homeless was used as an example. Another example of a type of support was admission to a nursing home. Participants suggested changing these examples in, for instance, lots of noises in the environment or inappropriate lighting.

The results of the panel group discussion were used to prepare a draft version of a tool that could be incorporated in the care programme for the detection of unmet needs in nursing home residents with young-onset dementia. The draft version, which covered 17 different areas of needs, was tested with people with young-onset dementia, their primary caregivers and the professional caregivers involved with their care. Four nurses administered the adapted CANE to eight people with young-onset dementia with less advanced dementia and relatively intact disease awareness and eight family caregivers of institutionalised people with young-onset dementia with moderate to advanced dementia.

People with young-onset dementia and their primary caregivers involved in the pilot found the tool relevant. It helped them think and talk about topics. The examples provided new insights into care options that were available to them. They also indicated that use of the instrument would be likely to improve the collaboration between paid and family caregivers, and they believed this to be very important to provide good-quality care. People with dementia and their caregivers in the pilot stated that the questions were clear. However, family caregivers felt that it is difficult for a caregiver to answer some of the questions when the person has advanced dementia. They stated that this was caused by the lack of communicative abilities of the person with dementia.

Nurses in the pilot stated that although administering the tool was perceived as time-consuming, it was feasible to use the tool in day-to-day practice. The nurses felt that the answers of the people with young-onset dementia and the family caregivers were very valuable. They explained that this information was helping them to get to know the residents and better understand their behaviour, especially in people who were recently admitted to the nursing home. The examples to identify needs and types of support to meet unmet needs were clear and provided useful starting points for possible interventions targeting unmet needs. The nurses mentioned that if no family caregiver was available, the tool could also be administered to another paid caregiver who had regular contact with the resident in the past month. The nurses, people with young-onset dementia and family caregivers participating in the pilot indicated that the draft version of the instrument was complete and that no changes or additions were necessary. They all stated that it is important to preserve the strength of the original CANE to investigate the needs from different perspectives: especially the family caregivers' and also formal caregivers' perspectives. Also, the advantage of the CANE in distinguishing between needs for which sufficient support is available and needs that are still unmet should be preserved.

The results of this small pilot study raise some interesting issues. First of all, although some alterations were made to the CANE for the particular purpose of use of the instrument in the care programme, the CANE appears to be a complete and thorough instrument that can also be used with younger people living with dementia. The results of the pilot study also underline that the setting and specific context in which the instrument is used should always be considered. Although needs occur in the same domains as in older people for younger individuals residing in nursing homes, the context of specific needs within specific domains and the types of possible support to meet unmet needs might differ. For example, people with young-onset dementia and older people both need appropriate daytime activities, but the types of daytime activities they prefer might be very different. The systematic assessment of these specific needs and types of support available were perceived as very valuable by both people with young-onset dementia in the pilot study and their paid and family caregivers. The study provides new insights to improve quality of care and improves collaboration between formal and informal caregivers. This suggests that the periodic assessment of the needs of people living with young-onset dementia should become part of common clinical practice. The tool developed in the BEYOND II study could be a promising starting point.

8.7 Conclusion

As we have seen, the number of studies addressing the needs of young people living with dementia and their family members are relatively scarce. Most often these studies rely on open interviews with caregivers of people with young-onset dementia and in some cases young people with dementia themselves. People with young-onset dementia consider themselves to be distinct from older individuals with dementia. The impact of living with dementia at a younger age should not be underestimated with regard to both the person with dementia and other family members. A family-oriented approach in healthcare provision is needed to allow for a better fit between the needs of these families and healthcare services. The results of the pilot study discussed in this chapter underline the importance of a systematic approach in the exploration of (unmet) needs in clinical practice and the possible resulting benefits.

References

1. Koopmans R, Rosness T. Young onset dementia: What does the name imply? *International Psychogeriatrics* 2014; **26**(12):1931–3.

2. Rabanal LI, Chatwin J, Walker A, et al. Understanding the needs and experiences of people with young onset dementia: A qualitative study. *BMJ Open* 2018; **8**(10):1–9.

3. Chemali Z, Schamber S, Tarbi E, et al. Diagnosing early onset dementia and then what? A frustrating system of aftercare resources. *International Journal of General Medicine* 2012; **5**:81–6.

4. Withall A, Draper B, Seeher K, Brodaty H. The prevalence and causes of younger onset dementia in Eastern Sydney, Australia. *International Psychogeriatrics* 2014; **26**(12):1955–65.

5. Kvello-Alme M, Brathen G, White LR, Sando SB. The prevalence and subtypes of young onset dementia in central Norway: A population-based study. *Journal of Alzheimer's Disease* 2019; **69**(2):479–87.

6. Mendez MF. The accurate diagnosis of early-onset dementia. *International Journal of Psychiatry in Medicine* 2006; **36**(4):401–12.

7. van Vliet D, de Vugt ME, Bakker C, et al. Time to diagnosis in young-onset dementia as compared with late-onset dementia. *Psychological Medicine* 2013; **43**(2):423–32.

8. Draper B, Cations M, White F, et al. Time to diagnosis in young-onset dementia and its determinants: The INSPIRED study. *International Journal of Geriatric Psychiatry* 2016; **31**(11):1217–24.

9. Kelley BJ, Boeve BF, Josephs KA. Cognitive and noncognitive neurological features of young-onset dementia. *Dementia and Geriatric Cognitive Disorders* 2009; **27**(6):564–71.

10. van Vliet D, de Vugt ME, Bakker C, et al. Caregivers' perspectives on the pre-diagnostic period in early onset dementia: A long and winding road. *International Psychogeriatrics* 2011; **23**(9): 1393–404.

11. Carter JE, Oyebode JR, Koopmans R. Young-onset dementia and the need for specialist care: A national and international perspective. *Aging & Mental Health* 2018; **22**(4):468–73.

12. Bakker C, de Vugt ME, van Vliet D, et al. The use of formal and informal care in early onset dementia: Results from the NeedYD study. *American Journal of Geriatric Psychiatry* 2013; **21**(1):37–45.

13. Harris PB, Keady J. Selfhood in younger onset dementia: Transitions and testimonies. *Aging & Mental Health* 2009; **13**(3):437–44.

14. Sperlinger D, Furst M. The service experiences of people with presenile dementia: A study of carers in one London borough. *International Journal of Geriatric Psychiatry* 1994; **9**(1):47–50.

15. van der Roest HG, Meiland FJ, Maroccini R, et al. Subjective needs of people with dementia: A review of the literature. *International Psychogeriatrics* 2007; **19**(3):559–92.

16. Bakker C, de Vugt ME, van Vliet D, et al. The relationship between unmet care needs in young-onset dementia and the course of neuropsychiatric symptoms: A two-year follow-up study. *International Psychogeriatrics* 2014; **26**(12): 1991–2000.

17. van Rijn A, Meiland F, Droes RM. Linking DemenTalent to meeting centers for people with dementia and their caregivers: A process analysis into facilitators and barriers in 12 Dutch meeting centers. *International Psychogeriatrics* 2019; **31**(10):1433–45.

18. van Vliet D, de Vugt ME, Kohler S, et al. Awareness and its association with affective symptoms in young-onset and late-onset Alzheimer disease: A prospective study. *Alzheimer Disease and Associated Disorders* 2013; **27**(3):265–71.

19. Williams T, Cameron I, Dearden T. From pillar to post: A study of younger people with dementia. *Psychiatric Bulletin* 2001; **25**(10):384–7.

20. Ducharme F, Kergoat MJ, Coulombe R, et al. Unmet support needs of early-onset dementia family caregivers: A mixed-design study. *BMC Nursing* 2014; **13**(1):1–10.

21. Cations M, Withall A, Horsfall R, et al. Why aren't people with young onset dementia and their supporters using formal services? Results from the INSPIRED study. *PloS One* 2017; **12**(7):1–10.

22. Millenaar JK, Bakker C, van Vliet D, et al. Exploring perspectives of young-onset dementia caregivers with high versus low unmet needs. *International Journal of Geriatric Psychiatry* 2017.

23. Bakker C, de Vugt ME, van Vliet D, et al. Predictors of the time to institutionalization in young- versus late-onset dementia: Results from the Needs in Young-Onset Dementia (NeedYD) study. *Journal of the American Medical Directors Association* 2013; **14**(4):248–53.

24. Millenaar JK, van Vliet D, Bakker C, et al. The experiences and needs of children living with a parent with young onset dementia: Results from the NeedYD study. *International Psychogeriatrics* 2014; **26**(12): 2001–10.

24a. Bruinsma J, Peetoom K, Bakker C, Boots L, Millenaar J, Verhey F, de Vugt M. Tailoring and evaluating the web-based 'partner in balance' intervention for family caregivers of persons with young-onset dementia. Internet Interventions. **25**:2021:100390.

25. Gelman C, Rhames K. 'I have to be both mother and father': The impact of young-onset dementia on the partner's parenting and the children's experience. *Dementia* 2020; **19**(3):676–90.

26. Sikes P, Hall M. It was then that I thought 'Whaat? This is not my Dad': The implications of the 'still the same person' narrative for children and young people who have a parent with dementia. *Dementia* 2018; **17**(2):180–98.

27. van Duinen-van den IJCL, Appelhof B, Zwijsen SA, et al. Behavior and Evolution of Young-Onset Dementia Part 2 (BEYOND II) study: An intervention study aimed at improvement in the management of neuropsychiatric symptoms in institutionalized people with young onset dementia. *International Psychogeriatrics* 2018; **30**(3):437–46.

Needs of Older People in Long-Term Care Settings

Justyna Mazurek, Dorota Szcześniak and Joanna Rymaszewska

Key Points

- There are significant risk factors for long-term care, which are age, gender, marital status, health and family history.
- Functional status and depressive symptoms are associated factors for perceived met and unmet needs among people living in long-term care settings.
- Despite many years of research, long-term care systems focus primarily on the physical difficulties of older patients, neglecting their psychosocial needs.
- Older people with dementia living in long-term care settings report fewer total needs than informal carers and more total and unmet needs than people without dementia.
- Staff members of care homes report more met and fewer unmet needs than older people with dementia.
- Older people with dementia usually report unmet needs in the areas of daytime activities, psychological distress, company and memory.
- Generally, in people with dementia, most unmet needs are associated with the poorest outcome measured (cognitive deficit, depressive symptoms, functional state, behavioural and psychological symptoms).
- The needs of institutionalised older people with dementia remain under-diagnosed and untreated.

9.1 Introduction

Rapid population aging which is the result of increasing longevity and declining fertility rates generates challenges that will require adjustments to the long-term care system. The institutionalisation rates increase dramatically with age. As little as 2% of the older population aged 65 to 74 years remains in nursing homes compared to 6% of the older population aged 75 to 84 years and 23% of those aged 85 or over.[1] These trends entail significant challenges for both the health and social sectors. However, it should be highlighted that the challenge is even greater when care of the quality of services offered is taken into consideration.

There are many definitions for long-term care in the literature. The National Institute of Aging emphasised that long-term care 'involves a variety of services designed to meet a person's health or personal care needs'.[2] These services pay special attention to independence and safety of people who can no longer perform everyday activities on their own. According to the World Health Organisation, the goal of long-term care systems is 'to ensure that an individual who is not fully capable of long-term self-care can maintain the best possible quality of life, with the greatest possible degree of independence, autonomy, participation, personal fulfilment and human dignity'.[3] Long-term care institutions refer to nursing and residential care facilities which provide accommodation and long-term care as a package. They include specially designed institutions of hospital-like settings where the predominant service component is long-term care and the services are provided for people with moderate to severe functional restrictions.

Older people enter 24-hour assisted living because support for their complex needs can no longer be provided in the community. The needs of older people living in long-term care settings are greater than for people staying in sheltered accommodation[4] or participating in day hospitals[5] and primary care.[6] The number of individuals with dementia who require residential care is substantial.[7] Older people with coexisting cognitive decline that remain in long-term care setting are at risk of having their needs ignored. The decisions are often made on their behalf by care home staff and/or informal carers or other people. Nevertheless, in fact, many older people are able to report their unmet and met needs despite suffering from moderately severe dementia.[8]

Unmet needs lead to a decreased quality of life, increased mental health problems and dissatisfaction with the services or even frustration or abuse of the older person.[9] The accurate assessment of these people is an important component of effective care delivery, particularly in institutionalised care. Moreover, such assessments can be acknowledged as better predictors of the worst prognostic outcomes than the usual applied measures of functional or cognitive decline.[10] It should be emphasised that institutionalisation rates increase when the dependency levels and needs of older people become too complex or too costly to be met at home or satisfied by available community services. In this context, higher demands are imposed on nursing homes and other long-term care facilities as their residents are becoming older, frailer and more dependent because of their physical and cognitive impairments.[11]

9.2 Needs of Older People in Long-Term Care Settings

Can we assume that there is a profile of a person who will need long-term care? Experience and practice emphasise that there are significant risk factors for long-term care, which are age, gender, marital status, health and family history (see Figure 9.1). This information at the very beginning determines the image of the person who will benefit from this type of support. Thus, it will probably be related to people vulnerable to a lack of psychosocial but also health-related needs from the start.

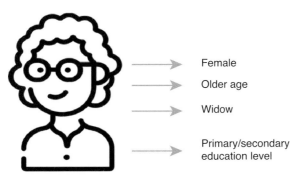

Female

Older age

Widow

Primary/secondary education level

Figure 9.1 Profile of an older person staying in a long-term care setting

This assumption is consistent with the results of many studies related to the needs assessment. Overall, older adults living in long-term care units had a higher number of needs; however, according to many studies, most of them were met especially in the environmental and physical domains.[9,12–14] This finding sounds very optimistic, and it indicates the adequacy of the proposed care. However, it is interesting to note that people with a lower Barthel Index and those with more depressive symptoms reported a greater number of needs overall, but these variables were not related to more unmet needs in some studies.[12] There are also studies which point out that the presence of unmet needs is associated with an increased cognitive and functional decline as well as with more depressive symptoms.[4,9,14,15] On the contrary, there are reports which emphasise that a worse functional status, higher level of cognitive impairment and more depressive symptoms are related to a higher level of met needs.[16] This last observation emphasises that when the patients' needs are clearly visible, any difficulties related to health can be considered as such; either somatic or mental, they will be taken into account and addressed properly in long-term care settings. This is in line with the work of German researchers, who pointed out that the long-term care system focuses primarily on the physical difficulties of older patients, neglecting their psychosocial needs.[17] This conclusion therefore reinforces the importance of assessing and analysing psychosocial needs.

Studies from various countries indicate that in long-term care it is important to pay attention to areas of needs which, despite many years of research, remain unmet. One of these is psychosocial needs, such as daytime activities, company, intimate relationships and psychological distress.[8,9,11] Moreover, research conducted in Poland indicates that the discrepancies between residents and staff members are visible in the number of unmet needs reported in relation to company and also psychological distress.[18,19] Staff members seem to be less aware of these unmet needs in comparison to users. Additionally, users frequently reported unmet needs in the area of daytime activities, eyesight/hearing/communication, information and intimate relationships, and similar conclusions were reported by Orrell et al.[8] An in-depth analysis of the users' perspective highlighted the lack of stimulating activities in the daily routine and the absence of more structured opportunities for social contacts. Bearing this in mind, these findings convey an important message concerning the significance of effective management of psychosocial needs' evaluation as well as interventions/programmes focused mainly on psychological and, what is more, also on social aspects of daily life.

Our conclusions on the research carried out so far on the assessment of needs fit perfectly into the constantly modified concept of health, which in 1948 was defined as 'a state of full physical, mental and social well-being and not just the lack of illness or disability'.[20] However, nowadays it has been enriched with a more holistic and dynamic understanding that promotes social aspects. According to Vernooij-Dassen et al.[21] the social health concept refers to the umbrella term related to human capacities to participate in social life with dignity and reciprocity. Therefore, all our activities related to the increase in the quality of services provided in long-term care units should also enable meeting the psychosocial needs of residents on an equal basis with the others.

9.3 Needs of Older People with Dementia in Long-Term Care Settings

Orrell et al.[8] compared the ratings of the needs of older people with dementia living in care homes, as assessed by the older person themselves, a family caregiver, and the staff of the care home. The authors showed that the staff reported more needs as met and fewer needs as unmet in many areas compared to the older people with dementia. The mean number of the needs identified by the older person with dementia was 10.21, by informal carers 14.49 and by staff 14.99. The users rated fewer needs met than carers and staff and a significantly higher average level of unmet needs for daytime activities and company.[8]

Van der Ploeg et al.[13] published a comparison between the care needs reported by older people with and without dementia in residential settings. They showed that older people with dementia reported fewer needs in total than their informal carers and more total and unmet needs than residents without dementia. The average number of needs was lower than in other studies (7.8 in total and 0.4 unmet needs).[13] Different results were obtained by Hancock et al.[9] They showed that unmet needs are associated with anxiety and depression, as well as with younger age and having resided in the care home for a shorter period of time, but not with the severity of dementia or level of dependency. The average number of needs

identified in the older people with dementia in residential care was 16.5, and 4.4 of them remained unmet (most commonly for stimulating daytime activities, psychological distress, memory and sensory problems and company). In a cluster randomised, controlled trial on the same group of older people with dementia, Orrell et al.[22] showed that after a 20-week follow-up intervention period (prioritisation of intervention, names of contact people and review dates, one hour per week), the unmet needs were reduced by 3.1 compared to a reduction of 0.7 in the control group without intervention. In the intervention group, the unmet needs were reduced particularly in four areas: eyesight/hearing, mobility, drugs and psychological distress. However, neither the level of quality of life nor depression nor dependency nor cognition improved in the intervention homes compared to the control homes that received care as usual.[22]

Ferreira et al.[11] found that there is a statistically significant negative correlation between Mini-Mental State Examination score and unmet, met and global needs. For people with cognitive decline, the mean number of unmet needs identified was four and included the areas of daytime activities, memory and psychotic symptoms. The authors also analysed data in order to compare unmet needs with severity stages of dementia. People in early stages had more unmet needs in daytime activities, eyesight/hearing and psychological distress, whereas older people in moderate stage presented more unmet needs in the areas of memory, psychotic symptoms and behaviour. Among the older people with severe dementia, daytime activities, memory and eyesight/hearing were the most frequently rated unmet needs.[11]

A much higher average level of total (20.4) and unmet (17.8) needs in older people with dementia living in long-term care institutions was obtained by Roszmann et al.[23] By contrast, similar to data from other authors, physical health needs were generally met, whereas there was a very high rate of unmet needs in the areas of emotional life and social interactions. The patients' four most frequently identified unmet needs were memory, psychological distress, intimate relationships, company and food.

9.4 Conclusion

The needs assessment has become a central issue following the growing recognition that it could lead to a more appropriate and effective provision of care.

The Camberwell Assessment of Need for the Elderly (CANE) is an effective method for identifying (un)met needs in older people living in long-term care institutions, as well as for those with dementia. On the basis of the studies that have been carried out so far, it can be concluded that systematic assessment may have led to a reduction in older people's unmet needs. Placing an emphasis on older people with and without dementia who live in long-term care setting will enhance the person's sense of identity, importance and quality of life.[8]

Long-term care settings seem to be better at meeting environmental and physical needs. The needs in the areas of daytime activities, company, memory and psychological distress remain unmet in institutionalised care settings.

The users' views on their needs should be taken into consideration even when the person is living with dementia in long-term care setting. People with dementia are often able to provide information regarding their needs, which is in line with the assumption that we should listen to every voice, especially the one of the people in question. Internationally, there is a drive to involve patients in health research, which is described as 'doing research with or by the patient rather than to, about, or for them'. This idea is particularly significant in the area of dementia and should be promoted not only in research but also in practice. The CANE provides a ready-made solution. It is known that to depend only on the assessment made by formal or informal carers may lead to an underestimation of unmet needs of older people. Even when older people have difficulties with verbal communication, staff members and informal carers should look out for nonverbal cues.[8] Staff members may need further education, appropriate training and support on how to recognise needs and solve older people's problems because people with dementia may not recall having certain needs or may have forgotten some of the services provided. Formal carers (staff) in long-term care settings may want to consider discussing care needs with both the older people themselves and their informal carers and integrate these reports.

Older people with dementia living in long-term care settings report fewer total needs than informal carers and more total and unmet needs than people without dementia, whereas the staff members of care homes report more met and fewer unmet needs than older people with dementia. This result may be understood as a lack of knowledge or skills to identify the unmet needs in this population. On the one hand, these differences could be due to the fact that the needs are underreported by older people with dementia. On the other hand, informal carers may overestimate the (un)met needs of their relatives with dementia.

References

1. Doty P, Liu K, Wiener J. An overview of long-term care. *Health Care Financing Review* 1985; **6**(3):69–78.

2. National Institute on Aging. Long-term care: What is long-term care? U.S. Department of Health and Human Studies, Washington, DC; 2017. Available at www.nia.nih.gov/health/what-long-term-care (accessed 15 January 2020).

3. World Health Organization, Department of Health Promotion. Health and aging discussion paper. WHO, Geneva; 2002. Available at https://apps.who.int/iris/handle/10665/66682 (accessed 15 January 2020).

4. Field E, Walker M, Orrell M. The needs of older people living in sheltered housing. In Orrell M, Hancock G (eds.), *CANE: Camberwell Assessment of Needs for the Elderly*. London: Gaskell; 2004:35–44.

5. Ashaye OA, Livingston G, Orrell M. Does standardized needs assessment improve the outcome of psychiatric day hospital care for older people? A randomised, controlled trial. *Aging & Mental Health* 2003; 7:195–9.

6. Walters K, Iliffe S, Tai SS, Orrell M. Assessing needs from patient, carer and professional perspectives: The Camberwell Assessment of Need for Elderly people in primary care. *Age & Ageing* 2000; **29**:505–10.

7. Kasper JD, Freedman VA, Spillman BC, Wolff JL. The disproportionate impact of dementia on family and unpaid caregiving to older adults. *Health Affairs (Millwood)* 2015; **34**(10):1642–9.

8. Orrell M, Hancock GA, Liyanage KC, et al. The needs of people with dementia in care homes: The perspectives of users, staff and family caregivers. *International Psychogeriatrics* 2008; **20**(5):941–51.

9. Hancock GA, Woods B, Hallis D, Orrell M. The needs of older people with dementia in residential care. *International Journal of Geriatric Psychiatry* 2006; **21**:43–9.

10. Gaugler JE, Kane RL, Kane RA, Newcomer R. Unmet care needs and key outcomes in dementia. *Journal of the American Geriatric Society* 2005; **53**(12):2098–105.

11. Ferreira AR, Dias CC, Fernandes L. Needs in nursing homes and their relation with cognitive and functional decline, behavioral and psychological symptoms. *Frontiers in Aging Neuroscience* 2016; **8**(72):1–10.

12. Tobis S, Wieczorowska-Tobis K, Talarska D, et al. Needs of older adults living in long-term care institutions: An observational study using Camberwell Assessment of Need for the Elderly. *Clinical Interventions in Aging* 2018; **13**:2389–95.

13. van der Ploeg ES, Bax DM, Nijpels G, van Hout HP. A cross-sectional study to compare care needs of individuals with and without dementia in residential homes in the Netherlands. *BMC Geriatrics* 2013; **13**:1–8.

14. Mazurek J, Rymaszewska J, Lurbiecki J. Comparison of the needs of the elderly patients in care-rehabilitation centers in Wroclaw and in Hamburg. *Advances in Rehabilitation* 2012; **26**(2):15–21.

15. Mazurek J, Szcześniak D, Urbańska KM, et al. Met and unmet care needs of the elderly with dementia living at home: Personal and informal carers' perspectives. *Dementia (London)* 2019; **18**(6): 1963–75.

16. Szczepańska-Gieracha J, Mazurek J, Kropińska S, et al. Needs assessment of people 75+ living in a nursing home or family home environment. *European Geriatric Medicine* 2015; **6**(4):348–53.

17. Richter D, Lowens S, Liekenbrock A. Need for psychosocial nursing care in a psychogeriatric nursing home. *Zeitschrift für Gerontologie + Geriatrie* 2000; **33**(1):17–23.

18. Talarska D, Wieczorowska-Tobis K, Kropińska S, et al. Care needs assessment in institutionalized elderly individuals based on CANE questionnaire. *Geriatria* 2012; **6**:1–8.

19. Wieczorowska-Tobis K, Talarska D, Kropińska S, et al. The Camberwell Assessment of Need for the Elderly questionnaire as a tool for the assessment of needs in elderly individuals living in long-term care institutions. *Archives of Gerontology and Geriatrics* 2016; **62**:163–8.

20. World Health Organization (WHO). Constitution of the World Health Organization. In *Basic Documents*, 45 ed. (Supplement). Geneva: WHO; 2006:1–18. Available at www.who.int/governance/eb/who_constitution_en.pdf (accessed 15 January 2020).

21. Vernooij-Dassen M, Jeon YH. Social health and dementia: The power of human capabilities. *International Psychogeriatrics* 2016; **28**(5):701–3.

22. Orrell M, Hancock G, Hoe J, et al. A cluster randomised, controlled trial to reduce the unmet needs of people with dementia living in residential care. *International Journal of Geriatric Psychiatry* 2007; **22**:1127–34.

23. Roszmann A, Żuralska E, Sitek EJ, et al. Needs assessment of long term care institutions residents with dementia. *Acta Neuropsychologica* 2014; **12**(1): 65–72.

Chapter 10

Needs and Healthcare Costs in Old Age

An Application of the Camberwell Assessment of Need for the Elderly

André Hajek, Janine Stein and Hans-Helmut König

10.1 Introduction

In industrialised countries, it is very likely that there will be a sharp rise in the number of individuals in old age in the upcoming decades. Common characteristics of these individuals include multi-morbidity or frequent doctor visits which are obviously linked to increased healthcare costs.[1] Therefore, identifying the determinants associated with increased healthcare costs among individuals in old age is crucial. Knowledge regarding these factors can help to manage healthcare services.

A widely used framework for analysing healthcare use and costs is the model developed by Ronald Andersen.[2] This model distinguishes between predisposing characteristics (e.g., sex), enabling resources (e.g., health insurance status) and need factors. In most studies that analysed healthcare costs, needs-related variables include measures of morbidity or physical functioning rather than actual measures of needs.[3] This is also true for studies that used Andersen's model to determine the factors associated with healthcare use or costs in old age.[2,3] Thus, it remains unknown whether actual needs are associated with healthcare costs in old age.[4] The Camberwell Assessment of Need for the Elderly (CANE) is a measure of actual needs that is widely used in other fields such as social psychiatry or care-related research.[4,6]

In this chapter, we present an application of the CANE for analysing healthcare costs. To this end, cross-sectional data of the Late-Life Depression in Primary Care: Needs, Health Care Utilisation and Costs (AgeMooDe) study are used. After a short description of the methods, results are depicted. The results will be discussed before drawing some general conclusions.

10.2 Methods

10.2.1 Sample

Baseline data from the AgeMooDe study were used for this analysis. It is a multicenter prospective cohort study which took place in four large German cities (Mannheim, Hamburg, Leipzig and Bonn). General practitioners (GPs) submitted lists of patients aged 75 and over and marked individuals with a depression diagnosis. Inclusion criterion was one or more GP visits in the past six months. Exclusion criteria at baseline were as follows: poorly known by the GP, poor German language skills, presence of dementia and suffering from severe illness with death likely to be within three months. Participants who remained on the list were invited to take part in this study. For each patient diagnosed with depression, another participant (age ± 2 years, same sex) not diagnosed with depression was randomly selected from the list and invited to take part in the AgeMooDe study. This means that these two groups are similar with regard to socio-demographic characteristics and number.

At baseline, 1,356 patients were recruited. Of this number, trained staff interviewed 1,230 individuals at home (from May 2012 to December 2013). In our analytical sample, 1,095 individuals were included. Further details are given elsewhere.[7]

The Ethics Committees of all participating centres approved the study (Ethics approval Leipzig: 020–12–23012012). Written informed consent was obtained from all GPs and patients.

10.2.2 Dependent Variable: Healthcare Costs

In this study, a societal perspective was adopted to compute healthcare costs. More precisely, irrespective of whether costs were reimbursed or not, all costs were considered in this study. Because individuals were 75 years of age and older, indirect costs determined by productivity losses were not considered because individuals aged 75 years and older are usually not involved in paid work. First, healthcare use was reported by the individuals. Afterwards, these numbers were multiplied by corresponding unit costs. A specifically designed generic questionnaire for individuals in late life, the Questionnaire for Health-Related Resource Use in an Elderly Population (FIMA; outpatient physician and non-physician services, pharmaceuticals, hospital treatment and rehabilitations, medical devices and formal and informal nursing care), was used to collect data on the health-related resource use.[8] For these sectors, health-related resource units were recorded. The recall period ranged from seven days (pharmaceuticals; in order to document long-term medications) to six months (the remaining healthcare resources; to reduce the trade-off between capturing rare events and decrease recall bias). Finally, unit costs were used for each resource to monetarily value these units. In the case of informal care, the proxy good method was used (€18.47 per hour). In the case of pharmaceuticals, official data on pharmaceutical selling prices were used to determine a price. These prices were assigned to the pharmaceuticals.[9] Further details are given elsewhere.[10]

10.2.3 Independent Variables

In this work, the CANE (German-language version) served as independent variable of interest.[11] It was developed from the Camberwell Assessment of Need (CAN).[12] In sum, 26 sections are covered in the CANE. While 2 sections quantify the needs of the person's caregiver, 24 sections measure individual needs.[13] The 24 sections include four care categories ((1) psychological, e.g., psychological distress or memory; (2) physical, e.g., falls or self-care; (3) social, e.g., intimate relationships or daytime activities; (4) environmental, e.g., looking after home or accommodation).[14] We used the number of needs in total as well as the number of needs in the four categories as main independent variables in this study. The favourable psychometric properties of the CANE have been demonstrated.[15,16]

Based on the Andersen model,[2] covariates were selected. With regards to predisposing characteristics, the model was adjusted for age, sex, marital status (married and living together with spouse, others

[married but not living together with spouse, divorced, widowed, single]) and the educational level (Comparative Analysis of Social Mobility in Industrial Nations (CASMIN)[17] [low, middle, high]). With regards to enabling resources, health insurance status (statutory health insurance, private health insurance) was used. With regards to illness-level characteristics, the Mini-Mental State Examination (from 0 [worst] to 30 [best]) was used to assess cognitive impairment.[18] Furthermore, to measure co-morbidity, the chronic disease score (CDS; based on pharmaceuticals; sum of each weighted pharmaceutical) was used.[19] Good psychometric characteristics have been reported.[20]

10.2.4 Statistical Analysis

Total costs were estimated using generalised linear models (with log link and gamma distribution) taking into account the highly skewed distribution of positive values.[21] This model is conventionally used in this area.[22] Average marginal effects (AMEs) of all variables were computed and displayed. They offer the advantage of interpretability, which means that they reflect the change in the outcome measure (costs in euros) associated with a one-unit change of the explanatory variable (for continuous variables; for categorical variables, the difference to the reference category). The outcome measures considered in this work include total costs from a societal perspective. The level of significance was fixed at 5%. Stata 15.1 (Stata Corp., College Station, Texas, USA) was used to perform statistical analysis.

10.3 Results

10.3.1 Sample Characteristics

Sample characteristics (for our analytical sample, $n = 1,095$) are depicted in Table 10.1. Average age was 80.7 years (±4.5 years; 75–98 years). Of the individuals, 63% were female, 54.3% had a low education level and 45.6% were married, living together with spouse. The average total number of needs was 4.4 (±3.3; average number of environmental needs: 0.9 [±1.2]; average number of physical needs: 2.4 [±1.4]; average number of psychological needs: 0.5 [±0.7]; average number of social needs: 0.6 [±0.7]). The average total healthcare cost per capita for a six-month period was €2,879 (±€5,611). Further details are presented in Table 10.1.

Table 10.1 Sample Characteristics (n = 1,095)

Variables	Mean (SD)/n (%)
Age: mean (SD)	80.7 (4.5)
Sex: n (%)	
Men	405 (37.0)
Women	690 (63.0)
Education: n (%)	
Low	595 (54.3)
Middle	294 (26.9)
High	206 (18.8)
Marital status: n (%)	
Married, living together with spouse	499 (45.6)
Other (married, living separated from spouse; single; divorced; widowed)	596 (54.4)
Health insurance: n (%)	
Private health insurance	48 (4.4)
Statutory health insurance	1,047 (95.6)
Cognitive impairment (Mini-Mental State Exam): mean (SD)	27.3 (2.4)
Co-morbidity (chronic disease score): mean (SD)	5.0 (3.0)
CANE: Number of needs (total): mean (SD)	4.4 (3.3)
CANE: Number of environmental needs: mean (SD)	0.9 (1.2)
CANE: Number of physical needs: mean (SD)	2.4 (1.4)
CANE: Number of psychological needs: mean (SD)	0.5 (0.7)
CANE: Number of social needs: mean (SD)	0.6 (0.7)
Total healthcare costs per capita (six-month period) in euros: mean (SD)	2,879.3 (5,611.6)

10.4 Regression Analysis

Results from multiple regression models (Table 10.2) are presented as AMEs of the independent variables on total healthcare costs. This means – and is worth repeating – that AMEs reflect the change in the outcome measure (costs in euros) associated with a one-unit change of the explanatory variable (for continuous variables; for categorical variables, the difference to the reference category). Adjusting for predisposing characteristics, enabling resources and several illness-level characteristics, the total number of needs was

associated with increased total healthcare costs (AME: €450.2; standard error [SE]: €57.3).

In addition, increased needs in all CANE categories were associated with increased total healthcare costs (environmental needs, AME: €1,259.0; SE: €181.0; physical needs, AME: €942.1; SE: €121.9; psychological needs, AME: €745.3; SE: €214.8; social needs: €777.4; SE: €167.3). With regards to covariates, only the co-morbidity was associated with the outcome variable in all models.

10.5 Discussion

While various other studies exist that investigated the determinants of healthcare use or costs in late life based on Andersen's model,[23,25] there is a lack of studies examining whether needs (in terms of CANE) are associated with healthcare costs among individuals in old age.[26] Therefore, our objective was to clarify whether these factors are associated cross-sectionally. After adjusting for predisposing characteristics, enabling resources and several illness-level characteristics, needs (total and each category) are independently associated with healthcare costs. Consequently, the study findings stress the importance of actual needs – quantified using the CANE – as determinants of healthcare costs.

Previous studies mainly demonstrated that increased illness-level characteristics are associated with increased healthcare use or costs.[3] However, they mainly focused on specific illnesses (e.g., stroke, cancer or hypertension) rather than assessing the needs of individuals. However, even after adjusting for numerous important covariates, this work shows that it is worth examining the link between actual needs (in terms of CANE) and healthcare costs in late life and consequently contributes to our understanding of this relationship.

In our view, it appears logical that increased actual needs are associated with higher healthcare costs because increased actual needs usually reflect, for example, illness symptoms. Moreover, increased needs (in terms of CANE) can also indicate difficulties in various other areas (such as distress or needs in intimate relationships), which can, in turn, increase the likelihood of doctor visits.[27] For example, needs in intimate relationships may, among others, reflect social isolation, which, in turn, has been linked to frequent attendance.[27] Because in the German healthcare system waiting times are quite short and most outpatient services are free of charge, these needs can be examined by the doctor with short or no waiting time.

Table 10.2 Determinants of Total Healthcare Costs (Societal Perspective): Results of Regression Analysis (Generalised Linear Models with Log Link and Gamma Distribution)

Independent Variables	(1) Total Costs (Societal Perspective)	(2) Total Costs (Societal Perspective)	(3) Total Costs (Societal Perspective)	(4) Total Costs (Societal Perspective)	(5) Total Costs (Societal Perspective)
Age	50.89†	33.37	58.92*	115.10**	99.69**
	(28.81)	(29.06)	(29.75)	(35.26)	(33.93)
Sex: Female (ref.: male)	348.33	169.01	323.10	435.44	503.89†
	(276.04)	(273.58)	(279.82)	(314.23)	(304.35)
Marital status: Other (ref.: married, living together with spouse)	-227.60	148.08	-260.81	68.04	-133.63
	(268.19)	(275.44)	(267.85)	(295.35)	(295.02)
Education: Middle (ref.: low)	-241.48	-209.94	-249.27	-600.34†	-460.16
	(252.14)	(264.55)	(240.74)	(319.17)	(303.71)
High	383.81	234.28	406.56	92.03	367.00
	(390.26)	(385.50)	(402.82)	(426.71)	(444.02)
Health insurance: Statutory health insurance (ref.: private health insurance)	-1,230.67**	-841.11†	-1,448.19***	-1,627.30**	-1,436.60**
	(445.91)	(486.40)	(436.73)	(515.43)	(477.36)
Cognitive impairment (MMSE)	-47.75	-32.28	-114.78†	-136.74*	-132.12*
	(55.42)	(53.24)	(60.74)	(69.69)	(65.40)
Chronic disease score (CDS)	193.40***	188.22***	185.31***	292.29***	276.15***
	(44.90)	(43.66)	(45.74)	(49.66)	(47.51)
CANE: Number of needs (total)	450.22***				
	(57.27)				
CANE: Number of environmental needs		1,259.03***			
		(180.95)			
CANE: Number of physical needs			942.06***		
			(121.93)		
CANE: Number of psychological needs				745.30***	
				(214.83)	
CANE: Number of social needs					777.43***
					(167.31)
Observations	1,095	1,095	1,095	1,095	1,095

Notes: Marginal effects are reported; standard errors in parentheses.

Some strengths and limitations are noteworthy. After adjusting for predisposing characteristics, enabling resources and several need factors, our study findings demonstrate that needs (quantified using the CANE) and healthcare costs are associated. The covariates were quantified using well-established scales. Data were drawn from a multicenter prospective cohort study. A societal perspective was adopted. The recall period was six months in order to tackle recall bias.[28] However, generalising our results to, for example, individuals residing in rural areas may be difficult.

10.6 Conclusion and Future Research

The CANE is widely used in other fields of research. We expected that need assessed by the CANE is also an important determinant of healthcare costs. Our aim was therefore to present an application of the CANE for analysing healthcare costs. Actually, the study findings emphasise the economic burden of increased actual needs among older adults. Thus, beyond commonly used need-related variables (e.g., morbidity or self-rated health), it may be worth including the CANE as a measure of actual needs in the Andersen model.

Future studies are required to shed more light on the link between actual needs (using the CANE) and healthcare costs. Thus, we hope that this work will inspire further research in this domain of CANE and healthcare costs. For example, given that data are available, future studies should draw on long-running panel studies. This may assist in clarifying whether long-term unmet needs are associated with marked increases in healthcare costs. Moreover, it may be worth investigating potential moderating variables (e.g., personality or coping strategies). For example, certain personality factors (such as neuroticism) or locus of control may moderate the link between actual needs and healthcare costs.[10,29]

Acknowledgements

This study was funded by the German Federal Ministry of Education and Research (Grant 01GY1155A) and the Federal Ministry of Health (Grant II A 5–2513 FSB 014). Publication was also supported by the study Healthy Aging: Gender-specific Trajectories into Latest Life (AgeDifferentDe), which was funded by the German Federal Ministry of Education and Research (Grants 01GL1714A, 01GL1714B, 01GL1714C, 01GL1714D).

The authors would like to thank all primary care patients and GPs for their participation and cooperation. Moreover, the authors would like to thank all members of the AgeMooDe study group, particularly the co-investigators Siegfried Weyerer, Wolfgang Maier, Martin Scherer, Birgitt Wiese and Steffi G. Riedel-Heller.

References

1. Smith J, Borchelt M, Maier H, Jopp D. Health and well-being in the young old and oldest old. *Journal of Social Issues* 2002; **58**(4):715–32.

2. Andersen RM. Revisiting the behavioral model and access to medical care: Does it matter? *Journal of Health and Social Behavior* 1995; **36**(1):1–10.

3. Babitsch B, Gohl D, von Lengerke T. Re-revisiting Andersen's behavioral model of health services use: A systematic review of studies from 1998–2011. *GMS Psycho-Social Medicine* 2012; **9**(11):1–15.

4. Alltag S, Stein J, Pabst A, et al. Unmet needs in the depressed primary care elderly and their relation to severity of depression: Results from the AgeMooDe study. *Aging & Mental Health* 2018; **22**(8):1038–45.

5. Kerpershoek L, de Vugt M, Wolfs C, et al. Needs and quality of life of people with middle-stage dementia and their family carers from the European Actifcare study: When informal care alone may not suffice. *Aging & Mental Health* 2018; **22**(7):897–902.

6. Tobis S, Wieczorowska-Tobis K, Talarska D, et al. Needs of older adults living in long-term care institutions: An observational study using Camberwell Assessment of Need for the Elderly. *Clinical Interventions in Aging* 2018; **13**:2389–95.

7. Stein J, Pabst A, Weyerer S, et al. The assessment of met and unmet care needs in the oldest old with and without depression using the Camberwell Assessment of Need for the Elderly (CANE): Results of the AgeMooDe study. *Journal of Affective Disorders* 2016; **193**:309–17.

8. Seidl H, Bowles D, Bock J, et al. FIMA – Questionnaire for health-related resource use in an elderly population: Development and pilot study. *Gesundheitswesen (Bundesverband der Ärzte des Öffentlichen Gesundheitsdienstes (Germany))* 2015; **77**(1):46–52.

9. Rote Liste. *Rote Liste Arzneimittelverzeichnis für Deutschland (einschließlich EU-Zulassungen und bestimmter Medizinprodukte)*. Frankfurt/Main: Rote Liste Service GmbH; 2011.

10. Hajek A, Bock J, König H. Which factors affect health care use among older Germans? Results of the German ageing survey. *BMC Health Services Research* 2017; **17**(1):1–8.

11. Dech H, Machleidt W. Relevance and applicability of the CANE in the German health care system. In Orrell H (ed.), *CANE: Camberwell Assessment of Need for the Elderly*. London: Gaskell; 2004:29–34.

12. Phelan M, Slade M, Thornicroft G, et al. The Camberwell Assessment of Need. *British Journal of Psychiatry* 1995; **167**(5):589–95.

13. Orrell M, Hancock G. CANE: Camberwell Assessment of Need for the Elderly. London: Gaskell; 2004.

14. Reynolds T, Thornicroft G, Abas M, et al. Camberwell Assessment of Need for the Elderly (CANE). *British Journal of Psychiatry* 2000; **176**(5):444–52.

15. Stein J, Luppa M, König H-H, Riedel-Heller SG. Assessing met and unmet needs in the oldest-old and psychometric properties of the German version of the Camberwell Assessment of Need for the Elderly (CANE): A pilot study. *International Psychogeriatrics* 2014; **26**(02):285–95.

16. Stein J, Luppa M, König H-H, Riedel-Heller SG. The German version of the Camberwell Assessment of Need for the Elderly (CANE): Evaluation of content validity and adaptation to the German-speaking context. *International Psychogeriatrics* 2015; **27**(11):1919–26.

17. Brauns H, Steinmann S. Educational reform in France, West-Germany, the United Kingdom and Hungary: Updating the CASMIN educational classification. *ZUMA-Nachrichten* 1999; **44**(23):7–44.

18. Folstein MF, Folstein SE, McHugh PR. 'Mini-Mental State': A practical method for grading the cognitive state of patients for the clinician. *Journal of Psychiatric Research* 1975; **12**(3):189–98.

19. Von Korff M, Wagner EH, Saunders K. A chronic disease score from automated pharmacy data. *Journal of Clinical Epidemiology* 1992; **45**(2):197–203.

20. Johnson RE, Hornbrook MC, Nichols GA. Replicating the chronic disease score (CDS) from automated pharmacy data. *Journal of Clinical Epidemiology* 1994; **47**(10):1191–9.

21. Moran JL, Solomon PJ, Peisach AR, Martin J. New models for old questions: Generalized linear models for cost prediction. *Journal of Evaluation in Clinical Practice* 2007; **13**(3):381–9.

22. Hohls J, Wild B, Heider D, et al. Association of generalized anxiety symptoms and panic with health care costs in older age: Results from the ESTHER cohort study. *Journal of Affective Disorders* 2019; **245**:978–86.

23. Hajek A, Bock J-O, Saum K-U, et al. Frailty and healthcare costs: Longitudinal results of a prospective cohort study. *Age & Ageing* 2017; **47**(2):233–41.

24. Hajek A, Brettschneider C, Eisele M, et al. Correlates of hospitalization among the oldest old: Results of the AgeCoDe–AgeQualiDe prospective cohort study. *Aging Clinical and Experimental Research* 2019; **32**:1295–301.

25. Hohls JK, König H-H, van den Bussche H, et al. Association of anxiety symptoms with health care use and costs in people aged 85 and over. *International Journal of Geriatric Psychiatry* 2019; **34**(5):765–76.

26. Hajek A, Brettschneider C, Scherer M, et al. Needs and health care costs in old age: A longitudinal perspective. Results from the AgeMooDe study. *Aging & Mental Health* 2020; **24**(10):1763–8.

27. Cruwys T, Wakefield JR, Sani F, et al. Social isolation predicts frequent attendance in primary care. *Annals of Behavioral Medicine* 2018; **52**(10):817–29.

28. Bhandari A, Wagner T. Self-reported utilization of health care services: Improving measurement and accuracy. *Medical Care Research and Review* 2006; **63**(2):217–35.

29. Bock JO, Hajek A, König HH. The longitudinal association between psychological factors and health care use. *Health Services Research* 2018; **53**(2):1065–91.

The Future of Needs Assessment Research

Juanita Hoe and Martin Orrell

11.1 Older People and Health

People are living longer, and the growth of the ageing population has led to an increase in demand for the use of health services. As life expectancy is extended, so the prevalence of long-term conditions and multimorbidity increases. While healthy ageing is achievable, the distribution of health depends on social and economic determinants, and improvements in health outcomes are associated with higher socioeconomic status.[1] Healthy ageing is linked to physical, mental, functional and social wellbeing but also depends on the role older people have in society and the reduction of age-discriminatory health inequalities.[2] Currently, ageing is associated with increased use of health services, but older people are generally considered lower priority for treatment and receive poorer-quality care.[3] Moreover, austerity measures over the last decade have led to a widening of social and economic inequalities, which have resulted in poorer health and increasing health inequality.[4] Constraints in spending on health and social care raise questions as to how health and social services will use the resources available to meet the needs of the older populations they serve.[5] Consequently, strategies for health must be adequately funded to counteract the significant impact of health inequalities on the needs of the older population and those with long-term conditions.[6]

Health needs encompass the wider social and environmental determinants of health, which include education, employment, housing, nutrition, lifestyle behaviours and social deprivation.[7] Needs assessment offers a systematic approach to assessing health needs and is used to identify inequalities in health and access to services and to determine priorities for the most effective use of resources.[8] It can include epidemiological, qualitative and comparative research methods for assessing how health and social services use their resources to meet the needs of the population and ensure that this is done in the most effective and efficient way.[9] To ensure that needs assessments are relevant for supporting health-related decision-making, research studies should focus on identifying the needs of targeted populations and include specific recommendations for policy based on the findings.[10]

11.2 Needs Assessment and the Health of Older People

The Camberwell Assessment of Need for the Elderly (CANE)[11] is a comprehensive and versatile needs assessment instrument that has been used to consistently measure the needs of older populations in a range of different contexts, which include public health, community and inpatient services for both generic health and mental health services and care-home settings. Application of the CANE within these settings is detailed in Chapter 1 of this book. Being widely translated into several languages shows the CANE's potential as an outcome measure for multinational psychosocial research, particularly in dementia.[12] The first INTERDEM manifesto outlines the need for better-quality research of psychosocial interventions for dementia that are driven by concept-informed outcome measures such as needs assessment to evaluate their effectiveness.[13] The design, evaluation and efficacy of psychosocial interventions for dementia have improved significantly over the past 20 years,[14] with interventions developed and tested for improving cognition,[15] activities of daily living,[16] mood,[17] behaviour[18] and carer wellbeing.[19] Furthermore, people with dementia are keen to be involved in the co-design of psychosocial interventions that meet their needs and allow them to feel safe to participate and to take risks, encourage social inclusion and promote dignity and wellbeing.[20] Additionally, the need for more research regarding psychosocial interventions for older people living at home, particularly those who are frail and housebound, has been identified.[21] The use of needs assessment was advocated for evaluating the effectiveness of care interventions delivered in the community. Individualised person-centred assessments have become the cornerstone of modern healthcare for older people, and these assessments need to be comprehensive and interdisciplinary to be effective.[22] The CANE is a useful tool for measuring need in older people with complex care and chronic health needs.[23] Furthermore, the inclusion of multiple perspectives in the CANE, particularly service user views, is seen as engaging older people with the needs assessment process and contributing to the validity of the instrument.[24] The review by Schmid et al.[25] assessing the validity, reliability and feasibility of 17 needs assessments for older people with cognitive impairment or dementia found that the CANE was the best instrument for comprehensively assessing the needs of older people with and without dementia.

11.3 Needs Assessment and Social Health

The second INTERDEM manifesto calls for research in dementia to focus on social health in order to bridge the gap between psychosocial and biomedical research using a framework of positive health.[26] Social health is viewed as connecting to both normality and neuropathology by accessing the cognitive reserve of people with dementia through promoting social inclusion,[27] as capacity in people with dementia can be influenced by using social resources to encourage maintaining independence and participation in social activities.[28] The concept of social health is important because across the numerous research studies that measure needs in older people using the CANE, the most consistently identified areas of unmet needs are in the social domain for the items daytime activities, company and intimate relationships (see Chapter 1). This includes both community and care-home settings and applies to those with and without dementia. Social isolation and loneliness are a risk factor for dementia and depression, which are influenced by living alone, lack of a spouse and social inactivity.[29,30] The *use it or lose it* theory posits that continued participation in social and cognitive activities helps build up brain reserve and can be influenced by environmental factors that promote physical activity and social engagement.[31] Developing integrated and person-centred approaches to health and social care systems is crucial for promoting better health, reducing

disease burden and responding to the needs of an ageing population.[32] Poor social health is a predictor for poor mental and physical health and increased mortality in older people; therefore, services that promote better heath, wellbeing and independence in older people can mitigate health inequalities and prevent or delay the need for institutional care.[6,33]

11.4 Needs Assessment and Technology

Technological advances have enabled care to be provided in different ways and may be a way to create more coherent and person-centred approaches for integrated health service delivery.[34] Actively engaging older people in the development of person-centred approaches to health service delivery ensures that they feel empowered by their inclusion in the design.[35] The use of assistive technology has been instrumental in supporting older people and those with long-term conditions to stay at home for longer.[36] Assistive technology enables people to live more healthy, productive, independent and dignified lives and reduces the need for health and social services support, carer involvement and long-term care.[37] Growing numbers of people aged 65 years and older have access to the internet, which enables increased social contact with family and friends and can be used for monitoring older people's health needs remotely.[38] In addition, older people are increasingly willing to do more for themselves and interact with services via technology.[5] Conversely, people with dementia often have difficulty using technology because the design of applications does not match their needs and capabilities, and they have not been involved in their conceptualisation.[39] There is, however, increasing evidence of the involvement of people with dementia in the exploratory and technical development phases of information technology applications, which they are enthusiastic about and feel empowered by their use.[40] People with dementia and family carers were involved in the development of a digital multifunctional device, the Cogknow Day Navigator, which was developed to support people with mild dementia in their daily lives, with memory, social contacts, daily activities and maintaining safety.[41] Needs assessment using the CANE was one of the outcomes measured in the project, although there was no change in the outcomes measured because of the short testing period and instability of the device. The inclusion of people with dementia and their carer's views, however, was seen to help improve the functionality of the device. For people with dementia and family carers, the most useful functions were help in cases of emergency, navigation support and the calendar function, which shows the potential for technology to provide personalised interventions that encourage independence and sustainability of daily activities and social needs.[42] Furthermore, there has been an increase in research related to dementia and the use of robots, which offer support with daily living activities, exercise and cognitive stimulation and provide companionship.[43] It would be of interest for needs assessment to be included in the evaluations of their use to help identify how effective robots are at meeting the needs of older people. Where technology is shown to be clinically useful and cost-effective, health and social care systems should expedite the assessment of its usefulness and scalability for practice.

11.5   Needs Assessment and Family Carers

Family carers look after someone with long-term physical or mental ill-health or disability, or who has care needs related to old age.[44] The number of people providing unpaid care globally to family members is rising, and in the United Kingdom there are currently estimated to be around 8.8 million carers.[45] Increasingly, the rights of carers are becoming enshrined in law in many countries,[46] and in the United Kingdom this includes the right to have an assessment of their need for support.[47] It is important that family carers are encouraged to balance their own needs with those of the person for whom they are caring, particularly as many are older and will have their own health needs.[48] To care for their family member safely and effectively, family carers should be offered an assessment of their own needs and be provided with information, support and care to meet those needs.[49]

Caring for an older person, especially one with dementia, can be very challenging and can have significant psychological and social consequences that affect the wellbeing of both the individual and their family. In particular, unmet needs for information and emotional and social support are associated with increased carer burden, depression and distress.[50,51] A review exploring how the needs of family carers are identified and assessed found only one validated assessment tool for measuring the needs of carers of people with dementia specifically, with several assessment tools combining carers' needs with assessment of the needs of the person with dementia.[52] This included the CANE, which includes two items for assessing carers' need for information and carers' psychological distress. Although the CANE is able to measure these needs in all carers of older people, the assessment of their needs is limited. Carers' ability to cope with caring is impacted by a range of physical and mental health, social and environmental factors, including their own physical health, mood, cognitive ability, alcohol or substance use, financial situation, employment needs, relationships and other caring responsibilities. In fact, there is a distinct lack of comprehensive needs assessment tools that can effectively measure the breadth of needs required and identify what support is required to enable the carer to care. If services are to support the carers of older people effectively, then the ability to assess and identify their needs and capacity to cope with caring is essential, and a robust assessment tool should be created that enables outcomes for carers to be reliably measured. This would allow for a more consistent approach to the assessment of carers' needs and enable health and social services to meet those needs.

11.6   Needs Assessment and Clinical Care

The applicability of the CANE for assessing the needs of older patients in routine clinical practice is apparent within the studies that have tested its acceptability with older populations across different clinical contexts and countries.[53–58] However, the CANE, as with other established needs assessments for older people,[59,60] has been viewed as cumbersome and time-consuming to complete.[61–63] The shortened version of the CANE was created as a more practical tool for use in clinical practice because it is quicker to complete yet retains the comprehensiveness and relevance of the fuller instrument as assessments are still made for each area of need. However, in some clinical areas, an even shorter version, such as the Senses (Vision and Hearing), Physical Ability (Mobility and Falls), Incontinence, Cognition and Emotional Distress (Depression and Anxiety) (SPICE), which was created for use in primary care settings, may be more appropriate.[64,65] The short version of the CANE has been used in several studies, and its use in clinical practice is advocated.[66,67] The fuller version of the CANE may be better for conducting service evaluations.

It has not been within the scope of this book to evaluate how the CANE has been used within clinical practice. Nonetheless, the CANE has received a lot of interest from practitioners, and the authors are aware that the instrument has been implemented clinically. Several professionals have contacted the authors seeking training on the use of the CANE or requested permission to include the tool within locally devised assessment packages for older people in health and social care services and the independent sector. However, the sustained use of the CANE within clinical areas is difficult to determine as the frequent reorganisation of UK health services means that changes in practice are commonplace, which impact on the structure of how care services and locally adopted practices are implemented. Furthermore, service evaluations undertaken locally to audit the needs of older populations are rarely published in the public domain. This is disappointing because the CANE is a valuable tool for identifying the needs of older people, particularly on entry into services, at times of crisis and during transitional phases, such as being discharged from hospital or when moving into long-term care. One of the possibilities to facilitate increased use of the CANE clinically could be to introduce an electronic version. With the advancement of information technology in the United Kingdom and other countries around the world, electronic health records have become firmly established in practice. However, the changes to data laws[68] and information governance[69] surrounding the use of patient information[70] means that introduction of an electronic version is unlikely. In addition, an electronic version of the CANE would need to be compatible for use with the multiple information technology systems that exist across health services, which is also improbable. It may be more feasible for local services to create their own electronic versions. Supporting older people with increasing levels of mental and physical frailty and complex health needs to remain at home for as long as possible is a national and global priority.[71–74] Therefore, the ability to provide reliable and comprehensive assessments of needs is essential. The evidence surrounding the use of the CANE, however, has shown its continued versatility and usefulness in assessing the met and unmet health and social needs of older people across a diverse range of clinical and non-clinical settings and patient groups.

11.7 Amendments to Update the CANE

Alongside the preparation of chapters for the second edition of the CANE, a team of three researchers led by one of the authors reviewed the prompts for each item used for applying the CANE in interviews. No changes were made to the key domains or items for needs, but some of the prompts were changed to reflect the changing needs of older people in modern times, and modifications were made to update some of the language used to more familiar modern-day terms. In addition, amendments were made to accommodate changes to legal terminology and the assessment of mental capacity and risk. Additions were also made to reflect the increased availability of therapeutic approaches for older people and specialist workers to support family carers. The term *insomnia* has also been added to the item physical care to reflect the prevalence of sleep disorders in older people. Also added were prompts that reflect the increasing vulnerability of older people to exploitation, poverty and homelessness and changes to welfare support. The most common changes related to adding prompts that take account of the increased use of assistive technology and accessibility of online resources, such as the use of social media, internet banking, online support and information.

11.8 Conclusion

Some of the priorities for future research regarding needs assessment have been outlined in this chapter and in other chapters within this book. These include to continue using needs assessment to identify gaps in service provision for older people so that services can be changed to meet those needs, to evaluate the effectiveness of psychosocial interventions and improve the social health of older people by increasing involvement in activities and reducing social isolation, to evaluate the effectiveness of assistive technology in supporting people to live independently at home, and to identify the needs of family carers to ensure that effective support is provided so that they can care for their family member better.

Ultimately, health inequalities lead to poorer healthcare, lower quality of life and less satisfaction with services. It is therefore paramount that we continue to assess the met and unmet needs of older people to ensure that services are able to meet the health needs of this population. Furthermore, meeting unmet need in one area can have a positive impact on the unmet needs in other areas, which can provide benefits for the individual. The CANE is a useful tool for assessing need, and needs assessment is an important outcome measure. However, needs assessment becomes irrelevant if actions are not undertaken to address the needs identified, and it is important that recommendations should be included for changes in policy to meet the unmet needs identified in research studies. Health policy and health services should be outcome driven, and it is important to show the benefits of new interventions for meeting the needs of the older population. Using the CANE is a very effective way to do this. Needs assessment facilitates improvements in health outcomes for older people, their quality of life and satisfaction with services. Individualised care depends on careful holistic assessment of older people and their situation, and evidence is now available regarding how such an assessment might best be approached.

References

1. Marmot M, Allen J, Bell R, et al. WHO European review of social determinants of health and the health divide. *Lancet* 2012; **380**(9846):1011–29.

2. Sadana R, Blas E, Budhwani S, et al. Healthy ageing: Raising awareness of inequalities, determinants, and what could be done to improve health equity. *Gerontologist* 2016; **56**(S2):S178–93.

3. Marmot M. *Review of Social Determinants and the Health Divide in the WHO European Region: Final Report.* Copenhagen: WHO Regional Office for Europe; 2013.

4. Marmot M. Health equity in England: The Marmot review 10 years on. *British Medical Journal* 2020; **368**: 1–4.

5. Ham C, Dixon A, Brooke B. *Transforming the Delivery of Health and Social Care.* Kings Fund Report. London: The Kings Fund; 2012.

6. Marmot M, Bell R. Fair society, healthy lives. *Public Health* 2012; **126**(Suppl. 1):S4–10.

7. Benzeval M, Bond L, Campbell M, et al. How does money influence health? Project report, Joseph Rowntree Foundation, York, UK; 2014.

8. Wright J, Williams R, Wilkinson JR. Development and importance of health needs assessment. *British Medical Journal* 1998; **316**(7140):1310–13.

9. Stevens A, Raftery J, Mant J, Simpson S. *Health Care Needs Assessment: The Epidemiologically Based Needs Assessment Reviews.* Abingdon, UK: Radcliffe Publishing; 2004.

10. Hensher M, Fulop N. The influence of health needs assessment on health care decision-making in London health authorities. *Journal of Health Services Research & Policy* 1999; **4**(2):90–5.

11. Reynolds T, Thornicroft G, Abas M, et al. Camberwell Assessment of Need for the Elderly (CANE): Development, validity and reliability. *British Journal of Psychiatry* 2000; **176**(5):444–52.

12. Moniz-Cook E, Vernooij-Dassen M, Woods R, et al. A European consensus on outcome measures for psychosocial intervention research in dementia care. *Aging & Mental Health* 2008; **12**(1):14–29.

13. Moniz-Cook E, Vernooij-Dassen M, Woods B, et al. Psychosocial interventions in dementia care research: The INTERDEM manifesto. *Aging & Mental Health* 2011; **15**(3):283–90.

14. Orrell M. The new generation of psychosocial interventions for dementia care. *British Journal of Psychiatry* 2012; **201**(5):342–3.

15. Spector A, Thorgrimsen L, Woods BO, et al. Efficacy of an evidence-based cognitive stimulation therapy programme for people with dementia: Randomised, controlled trial. *British Journal of Psychiatry* 2003; **183** (3):248–54.

16. Graff MJ, Vernooij-Dassen MJ, Thijssen M, et al. Community based occupational therapy for patients with dementia and their care givers: Randomised, controlled trial. *British Medical Journal* 2006; **333** (7580):1196–9.

17. Teri L, Gibbons LE, McCurry SM, et al. Exercise plus behavioral management in patients with Alzheimer disease: A randomized, controlled trial. *Journal of the American Medical Association* 2003; **290**(15):2015–22.

18. Livingston G, Barber J, Marston L, et al. Clinical and cost-effectiveness of the Managing Agitation and Raising Quality of Life (MARQUE) intervention for agitation in people with dementia in care homes: A single-blind, cluster-randomised, controlled trial. *Lancet Psychiatry* 2019; **6**(4): 293–304.

19. Livingston G, Barber J, Rapaport P, et al. Clinical effectiveness of a manual based coping strategy programme (START, STrAtegies for RelaTives) in promoting the mental health of carers of family members with dementia: Pragmatic randomised controlled trial. *British Medical Journal* 2013; **347**:1–14.

20. Øksnebjerg L, Diaz-Ponce A, Gove D, et al. Towards capturing meaningful outcomes for people with dementia in psychosocial intervention research: A pan-European consultation. *Health Expectations* 2018; **21**(6):1056–65.

21. de Rossi Figueiredo D, Paes LG, Warmling AM, et al. Multidimensional measures validated for home health needs of older persons: A systematic review. *International Journal of Nursing Studies* 2018; **77**:130–7.

22. Davis S, Dorevitch M, Garratt S. Person-centred comprehensive geriatric assessment. In: *Older People: Issues and Innovations in Care*. Sydney: Churchill Livingstone; 2009:168–88.

23. Foreman P, Thomas S, Gardner I. The review and identification of an existing, validated, comprehensive assessment tool. Report for the Department of Human Services, Lincoln Centre for Ageing and Community Care Research, Australian Institute for Primary Care at La Trobe University, Melbourne, Australia; 2004.

24. Moriarty J. Assessing the mental health needs of older people: Systematic review on the use of standardised measures to improve assessment practice. Social Care Workforce Research Unit Report, King's College, London; 2002.

25. Schmid R, Eschen A, Rüegger-Frey B, Martin M. Instruments for comprehensive needs assessment in individuals with cognitive complaints, mild cognitive impairment or dementia: A systematic review. *International Journal of Geriatric Psychiatry* 2012; **27** (4):329–41.

26. Vernooij-Dassen M, Moniz-Cook E, Verhey F, et al. Bridging the divide between biomedical and psychosocial approaches in dementia research: The 2019 INTERDEM manifesto. *Aging & Mental Health* 2020; 1–7.

27. Vernooij-Dassen M, Jeon YH. Social health and dementia: The power of human capabilities. *International Psychogeriatrics* 2016; **28** (5):701–3.

28. Huber M, Knottnerus JA, Green L, et al. How should we define health? *British Medical Journal* 2011; **343** (7817):1–3.

29. Sundström A, Adolfsson AN, Nordin M, Adolfsson R. Loneliness increases the risk of all-cause dementia and Alzheimer's disease. *Journal of Gerontology: Series B* 2020; **75**(5):919–26.

30. Sundström A, Westerlund O, Kotyrlo E. Marital status and risk of dementia: A nationwide population-based prospective study from Sweden. *British Medical Journal Open* 2016; **6**(1):1–7.

31. Scarmeas N, Stern Y. Cognitive reserve: implications for diagnosis and prevention of Alzheimer's disease. *Current Neurology and Neuroscience Reports* 2004; **4** (5):374–80.

32. World Health Organization (WHO). *Framework on Integrated, People-Centred Health Services*. Geneva: WHO; 2016.

33. Marmot M, Allen J, Bell R, et al. WHO European review of social determinants of health and the health divide. *Lancet* 2012; **380**(9846):1011–29.

34. Phanareth K, Vingtoft S, Christensen AS, et al. The Epital care model: A new person-centered model of technology-enabled integrated care for people with long term conditions. *Journal of Medical Internet Research* 2017; **6**(1):1–15.

35. Kayser L, Karnoe A, Duminski E, et al. A new understanding of health related empowerment in the context of an active and healthy ageing. *BMC Health Services Research* 2019; **19**(1):1–13.

36. World Health Organization (WHO). *Global Cooperation on Assistive Technology (GATE)*. Geneva: WHO; 2014.

37. World Health Organization (WHO). *Assistive Technology Fact Sheet*. Geneva: WHO; 2018.

38. Age UK. *Technology and Older People Evidence Review*. London: Age UK; 2010.

39. Hanson E, Magnusson L, Arvidsson H, et al. Working together with persons with early stage dementia and their family members to design a user-friendly technology-based support service. *Dementia* 2007; **6** (3):411–34.

40. Span M, Hettinga M, Vernooij-Dassen M, et al. Involving people with dementia in the development of supportive IT applications: A systematic review. *Ageing Research Reviews* 2013; **12**(2):535–51.

41. Meiland FJ, Bouman AI, Sävenstedt S, et al. Usability of a new electronic assistive device for community-dwelling persons with mild dementia. *Aging & Mental Health* 2012; **16**(5):584–91.

42. Meiland FJ, Hattink BJ, Overmars-Marx T, et al. Participation of end users in the design of assistive technology for people with mild to severe cognitive problems: The European Rosetta Project. *International Psychogeriatrics* 2014; **26**(5):769–79.

43. Cruz-Sandoval D, Morales-Tellez A, Sandoval EB, et al. Robot as therapy facilitator in interventions to deal with dementia-related behavioral symptoms. In *Proceedings of the 2020 ACM/IEEE International Conference on Human-Robot Interaction*. New York: Association for Computing Machinery; 2020:161–9.

44. Carers E. Embracing the critical role of caregivers around the world. White paper and action plan, Darmstadt, Germany; 2017.

45. Carers UK. State of caring: A snapshot of unpaid care in the UK. State of Caring Report, London; 2019.

46. Bouget D, Saraceno C, Spasova S. Towards new work-life balance policies for those caring for dependent relatives? In Vanhercke B, Sabato S, Bouget D (eds.), *Social Policy in the European Union: State of Play*.

Eighteenth annual report. Brussels: ETUI - European Trade Union Institute; 2017:155–7.

47. Her Majesty's Government. Care Act 2014 (c. 23). London: The Stationery Office (TSO); 2014.

48. Milne A, Hatzidimitriadou E, Chryssanthopoulou C, Owen T. Caring in later life: Reviewing the role of older carers. Help the Aged; 2001.

49. Department of Health. Caring about carers: A national strategy for carers. White paper, Department of Health, London; 1999.

50. Harland JA, Bath PA. Understanding the information behaviours of carers of people with dementia: A critical review of models from information science. *Aging & Mental Health* 2008; **12**(4):467–77.

51. Gaugler JE, Anderson KA, Leach CR, et al. The emotional ramifications of unmet need in dementia caregiving. *American Journal of Alzheimer's Disease & Other Dementias* 2004; **19**(6):369–80.

52. Novais T, Dauphinot V, Krolak-Salmon P, Mouchoux C. How to explore the needs of informal caregivers of individuals with cognitive impairment in Alzheimer's disease or related diseases? A systematic review of quantitative and qualitative studies. *BMC Geriatrics* 2017; **17**(1):1–8.

53. Fernandes L, Gonçalves-Pereira M, Leuschner A, et al. Validation study of the Camberwell Assessment of Need for the Elderly (CANE) in Portugal. *International Psychogeriatrics* 2009; **21**(1):1–9.

54. Park M, Kim SK, Jeong M, et al. Psychometric validation of the Korean version of the Camberwell assessment of need for the elderly in individuals with dementia. *Asian Nursing Research* 2018; **12**(2):106–12.

55. Stein J, Luppa M, König HH, Riedel-Heller SG. The German version of the Camberwell Assessment of Need for the Elderly (CANE): Evaluation of content validity and adaptation to the German-speaking context. *International Psychogeriatrics* 2015; **27**(11):1919–26.

56. Salehi R, Davatgaran K, Heidari M, et al. The psychometric properties of the Persian version of the Camberwell Assessment of Needs (CANE) for Iranian elderly people with mental disorders. *Iranian Journal of Ageing* 2018; **13**(2):168–81.

57. Greaves S, Bhat M, Regan C, et al. The unmet needs of referrals to old age psychiatry liaison services. *Psychogeriatria Polska* 2006; **3**(4):175–82.

58. Wieczorowska-Tobis K, Talarska D, Kropińska S, et al. The Camberwell Assessment of Need for the Elderly questionnaire as a tool for the assessment of needs in elderly individuals living in long-term care institutions. *Archives of Gerontology & Geriatrics* 2016; **62**:163–8.

59. Philp I. EASY-Care: A systematic approach to the assessment of older people. *Geriatric Medicine* 2000; **30**(5):15–19.

60. Carpenter GI. *InterRAI UK MDS Home Care Assessment Instrument for Community Care: User's Manual.* York, UK: InterRAIUK; 2002.

61. Murray J, Young J, Forster A. Measuring outcomes in the longer term after a stroke. *Clinical Rehabilitation* 2009; **23**(10):918–21.

62. Gonçalves-Pereira M, Fernandes L, Leuschner A, et al. Versão portuguesa do CANE (Camberwell Assessment of Need for the Elderly): Desenvolvimento e dados preliminares. *Revista Portuguesa de Saúde Pública* 2007; **25**(1):7–18.

63. Hoogendijk EO, Muntinga ME, van Leeuwen KM, et al. Self-perceived met and unmet care needs of frail older adults in primary care. *Archives of Gerontology and Geriatrics* 2014; **58**(1):37–42.

64. Iliffe S, Lenihan P, Orrell M, et al. The development of a short instrument to identify common unmet needs in older people in general practice. *British Journal of General Practice* 2004; **54**(509):914–18.

65. Balsinha C, Marques MJ, Gonçalves-Pereira M. A brief assessment unravels unmet needs of older people in primary care: A mixed-methods evaluation of the SPICE tool in Portugal. *Primary Health Care Research & Development* 2018; **19**(6):637–43.

66. Rymaszewska J, Kłak R, Synak A. Camberwell Assessment of Need for the Elderly (CANE): Badanie polskiej wersji narzędzia. *Psychogeriatria Polska* 2008; **5**(2):105–13.

67. Fink HA. Testing of the Camberwell Assessment of Need for the Elderly (CANE) in a German setting. Doctoral dissertation, Medical University, Berlin, Germany; 2011.

68. Regulation protection: General data protection regulation. Weston-super-Mare, UK: InTouch CRM; 2018. Available at www.intouchcrm.com/about-gdpr/ (accessed 27 July 2020).

69. National Health Service. *Encryption: Good Practice Guidance.* Leeds, UK: NHS; 2020. Available at https://digital.nhs.uk/services/data-and-cyber-security-protecting-information-and-data-in-health-and-care/cyber-anddata-security-policy-and-good-practice-in-health-and-care/encryption-guidance-forhealth-and-care-organisations (accessed 27 July 2020).

70. British Psychological Society. Electronic records guidance. BPS, Leeds, UK; 2019.

71. Department of Health. Prime Minister's challenge on dementia 2020: Implementation plan. Department of Health, London; 2015. Available at www.gov .uk/government/publications/challenge-on-demen tia-2020-implementation-plan.

72. House of Lords Select Committee on Public Service and Demographic Change. *Ready for Ageing Report*, vol. 2. London: The Stationery Office; 2013. Available at https://publications.parliament.uk/pa/ld201213/ ldselect/ldpublic/140/14002.htm (accessed 27 July 2020).

73. NHS England. Five-year forward view. NHS, London; 2014. Available at www.england.nhs.uk/five-year-forward-view/(accessed 27 July 2020).

74. World Health Organization (WHO). *Global Action Plan on the Public Health Response to Dementia 2017–2025*. Geneva: WHO; 2017.

Instructions for the CANE

CAMBERWELL
ASSESSMENT OF NEED
FOR THE ELDERLY

CANE

Version V

CODE	

Interviewee	Date	Interview Time
User		
Carer		
Staff		
Rater/Clinician		

Background Details
(please fill in blanks, or circle whichever applies)

CODE NUMBER: _____

Date of Birth: _____ AGE: _____(years)

SEX: male / female

ETHNICITY: Asian/ African/ African-American/ Black Caribbean / White/ Other_____

RELIGION: Christian/ Muslim/ Hindu/ Jewish/ Other_____

FIRST LANGUAGE : English/Other _____

MARITAL STATUS: single / married / divorced / separated / widowed

LIVING SITUATION: alone / with partner / with other relatives / with others

LIVING ENVIRONMENT: flat / house / sheltered / residential / nursing / other

PREVIOUS OCCUPATION (or partner's): _____

EDUCATION: _____(years)

CURRENT STATUS: in-patient / day-patient / community patient (Psychiatric / Geriatric/other)

MAIN DIAGNOSES (DSM-IV/ICD 10): _____
_____
_____
_____

CURRENT MEDICATION: _____
_____

DISEASE PREVENTION: (e.g. blood pressure/smoking/sleep pattern/exercise/health screening/vaccination)

_____

DOES THE PERSON HAVE A FAMILY CARER? yes / no

IS THE PERSON A FAMILY CARER? yes / no

The Camberwell Assessment of Need for the Elderly (CANE) is a comprehensive, person-centred needs assessment tool that has been designed for use with older people. It is suitable for use in a variety of clinical and research settings. The CANE has a person-centred approach which allows views of the professional, user and carer to be recorded and compared. The instrument uses the principle that identifying a need means identifying a problem plus an appropriate intervention which will help or alleviate the need. Therefore, the CANE models clinical practice and relies on professional expertise for ratings to be completed accurately. Professionals using the CANE need to have had training and experience working with older people and an adequate knowledge of clinical interviewing and decision-making. They should also have good working knowledge of the concepts of need, met need and unmet need. This knowledge can be gained with experience of the full CANE assessments and reference to the manual.

There are 24 topics relating to the user and two (A and B) relating to the carer. There are four columns to document ratings so that one or more of the user (U), staff member (S), carer (C) or rater (clinician/ researcher) (R) can each express their view. Note at the top of the column which person has been interviewed.

Section 1

This section aims to assess whether there is currently a need in the specific area. A *need* is defined as a problem with a potential remedy or intervention. Use the prompts below each area in italics on the record form to establish the user's current status with regards to the need area. If there has been a need, then assess whether it was met appropriately. Score each interviewee independently, even though their perceptions of need in each area may differ from those of others. The administrator should ask additional questions probing into the area until he or she can establish whether the person has a significant need that requires assistance and whether he or she is getting enough of the right type of help. Once this information has been gathered, a rating of need can be made. Judgement of rating in this section should be based on normal clinical practice. The CANE is intended to be a framework for assessment grounded in good professional practice and expertise. Although Section 1 in each problem area is the main section of interest to CANE administrators, it often cannot be rated until adequate information has been collected about the area. Indeed, some administrators have found it easier to rate Section 1 once information has been collected from Sections 2 to 5. When adequate information has been gathered, the rater should clearly be able to make a clinical judgement as to whether the area is a met need, an unmet need or is not a need for the person. Confusion with ratings can be avoided by not directly asking a closed question about whether there is a problem in a certain area (e.g., 'Do you have any problems with the food here?') because the person can answer 'No'. This response may then be mistaken as a 'No need', where in fact it is a 'Met need' because the person is assisted by someone else.

♦ *No need*: Score 0 there if there is no need in the area; then go on to the next page. In this situation, the user is coping well independently and does not need any further assistance. For example, the user has reported that they are successfully administering their own medication and do not have any problematic side effects. Or the staff member reports that the user appeared to be comfortable in his or her home environment and that no alterations to the building are needed or planned.

♦ *Met need*: Score 1 if the need is met or if there is a minor need requiring no significant intervention. A need is met when there is a mild, moderate or serious problem which is receiving an intervention that is appropriate and potentially of benefit. This category is also used for problems which would normally not be of clinical significance and would not require a specific intervention. For example, the user is receiving an assessment for poor eyesight or a district nurse is overseeing the administration of medications each day.

♦ *Unmet need*: Score 2 if the need is currently unmet. An unmet need is a serious problem requiring intervention or assessment, which is currently receiving no assistance or the *wrong* type or level of help, for example, if a staff member reported that the user was incontinent of large amounts of urine every night despite toileting twice during the night and that the use of pads and further assessment or an intervention was required, or a carer reported that the user had become very hard of hearing and had not received an assessment or suitable hearing aids.

♦ *Unknown:* Score 9 if the person does not know about the nature of the problems or about the assistance the person receives; then go on to the next page. Such a score may mean that further information is needed to make a rating.

For any topic, if Section 1 is rated as 1 or 2, complete Sections 2–4. If Section 1 for the topic is rated as 0 or 9, do not complete Sections 2–4 but go to the next topic area.

Section 2

This section asks about assistance from informal sources during the past month. Informal sources include family, friends or neighbours. Use the examples on the assessment form to prompt the interviewee. Score 1 when assistance is given very occasionally or infrequently. Score 2 when assistance is given more frequently or involves more time/effort. Score 3 when assistance is given daily or is intensive (e.g., long periods of respite). Score 4 when assistance is very intensive and/or daily (e.g., family lives with the user and gives them full assistance with most tasks). Score 9 if the interviewee is unsure of the level of assistance provided.

Section 3

i. This section asks whether the user receives any assistance from local services to help with the problem. These formal supports are defined above to include paid carers, residential care, long-term wards, formal respite, day-care centres, hospitals, community psychiatric nurses or other staff. Use the examples on the assessment form to prompt the interviewee. Score 1 for minimal support, occasional or light support. Score 2 for more regular assistance, maybe once a week or more significant support occasionally. Score 3 for specialist assistance, currently under assessment or more frequent assistance. Score 9 if the interviewee is unsure of the level of assistance provided.

ii. The second part to Section 3 asks what formal supports the interviewer feels the user *requires,* using the same scale as in part (i) of Section 3. This second part indicates under-met need, where the person is getting (part (i)) less than they require (part (ii)), or overprovision of need, where the person is getting (part (i)) a higher level of service than they require (part (ii)).

Section 4

i. This section asks whether the person feels that the user is receiving the right type of help with the problem. The answer to this question may have been obvious from the responses to the previous section, especially Section 1. However, if in doubt, ask more specifically. As well as highlighting unmet needs, this section can point out overprovision of needs, where the person reported that the user was receiving a higher level of assistance than they required.

ii. The second question in Section 4 asks about the user's satisfaction with the assistance they are receiving. Again, this may be obvious from prior responses, but please ask specifically.

Section 5

This section is for noting the individual details of the assessment and the details of the help the user receives and requires (particularly the nature of the unmet needs identified) in order to formulate an action plan. Problems with current interventions or care plans and plans in progress should also be documented in this section. Use codes to document which informant has provided the information (i.e., U = user; S = staff; C = carer; R = rater/professional). Users' perspectives on their expectations, personal strengths and resources should be noted here. Individual spiritual and cultural information should also be noted in this section. This information is vital for establishing an effective individualised care plan.

Scoring

It is to be noted that scoring is a secondary aspect of the CANE, as its primary purpose is to identify and assess individual unmet needs. The total CANE score is based on the rating of Section 1 of each of the 24 problem areas. The two areas (A and B) relating to carers' needs are not added into this total score. Count the total number of met needs (rated as a 1 in Section 1) out of a maximum of 24. Count the total number of unmet needs identified (rated as a 2 in Section 1) out of a maximum of 24. Count the total number of needs identified (rated as a 1 or 2 in Section 1) out of a maximum of 24. The raters' (clinicians or researchers) ratings are made based on all the information gathered through the assessment. Raters' ratings of Section 1 are used as the basis for total CANE scores.

1. ACCOMMODATION

ASSESSMENTS
user   carer   staff   rater

DOES THE PERSON HAVE AN APPROPRIATE PLACE TO LIVE?

What kind of home do you live in? Do you have any problems with accommodation?

0 = NO NEED   e.g. Has an adequate and appropriate home (even if currently in hospital). No need for assistance with accommodation

1 = MET NEED   e.g. Home undergoing adaptation/redecoration. Needs and is getting help with accommodation, e.g., in residential care, sheltered housing.

2 = UNMET NEED   e.g. Homeless, inappropriately housed or home lacks basic facilities such as water, electricity, heating or essential alterations. Person is facing eviction

9 = NOT KNOWN

IF RATED 0 OR 9 GO TO QUESTION 2

HOW MUCH HELP DOES THE PERSON RECEIVE FROM RELATIVES OR FRIENDS WITH THEIR ACCOMMODATION

0 = NONE

1 = LOW HELP   e.g. Occasionally does odd jobs concerning accommodation e.g., minor redecorations.

2 = MODERATE HELP   e.g. Substantial help with improving accommodation such as organising redecoration or specific adaptations. Repairs and maintenance

3 = HIGH HELP   e.g. Living with a relative because own accommodation is unsatisfactory.

9 = NOT KNOWN

HOW MUCH HELP DOES THE PERSON RECEIVE FROM LOCAL SERVICES WITH THEIR ACCOMMODATION?

HOW MUCH HELP DOES THE PERSON NEED FROM LOCAL SERVICES WITH THEIR ACCOMMODATION?

0 = NONE

1 = LOW HELP   e.g. Minor redecoration; Referral to housing agency/ assisted housing.

2 = MODERATE HELP   e.g. Major improvements; actively pursuing change in accommodation.

3 = HIGH HELP   e.g. Being rehoused; living in supported accommodation residential care, nursing home or continuing care hospital ward.

9 = NOT KNOWN

DOES THE PERSON RECEIVE THE RIGHT TYPE OF HELP WITH THEIR ACCOMMODATION? (0 = NO   1 = YES   9 = NOT KNOWN)

OVERALL, IS THE PERSON SATISFIED WITH THE AMOUNT OF HELP THEY ARE RECEIVING WITH ACCOMMODATION?
(0 = NOT SATISFIED   1 = SATISFIED   9 = NOT KNOWN)

COMMENTS

2. LOOKING AFTER THE HOME

ASSESSMENTS

user   carer   staff   rater

DOES THE PERSON HAVE DIFFICULTY IN LOOKING AFTER THEIR HOME?

Are you able to look after your household chores?
Does anyone help you?

0 = NO NEED — e.g. Independent in looking after the home, home may be untidy but kept basically clean.

1 = MET NEED — e.g. Limited in looking after home and has appropriate level of domestic help. Has private cleaner

2 = UNMET NEED — e.g. Not receiving appropriate level of domestic assistance. Home is a potential health/fire/escape hazard. Squalid - environmental cleaning team needed.

9 = NOT KNOWN

IF RATED 0 OR 9 GO TO QUESTION 3

HOW MUCH HELP DOES THE PERSON RECEIVE FROM RELATIVES OR FRIENDS WITH LOOKING AFTER THE HOME?

0 = NONE

1 = LOW HELP — e.g. Prompts or helps tidy up or clean occasionally.

2 = MODERATE HELP — e.g. Prompts or helps cleans at least once a week.

3 = HIGH HELP — e.g. Does most or all of the household tasks.

9 = NOT KNOWN

HOW MUCH HELP DOES THE PERSON RECEIVE FROM LOCAL SERVICES WITH LOOKING AFTER THE HOME?

HOW MUCH HELP DOES THE PERSON NEED FROM LOCAL SERVICES WITH LOOKING AFTER THE HOME?

0 = NONE

1 = LOW HELP — e.g. Prompting / supervision by staff.

2 = MODERATE HELP — e.g. Some assistance with household tasks.

3 = HIGH HELP — e.g. Majority of household tasks done by staff.

9 = NOT KNOWN

DOES THE PERSON RECEIVE THE RIGHT TYPE OF HELP WITH LOOKING AFTER THE HOME? (0 = NO   1 = YES   9 = NOT KNOWN)

OVERALL, IS THE PERSON SATISFIED WITH THE AMOUNT OF HELP THEY ARE RECEIVING WITH LOOKING AFTER THE HOME? (0 = NOT SATISFIED   1 = SATISFIED   9 = NOT KNOWN)

COMMENTS

3. FOOD

DOES THE PERSON HAVE DIFFICULTY IN GETTING ENOUGH TO EAT?

Are you able to prepare your own meals and do your own shopping?
Are you getting the right sort of food?

0 = NO NEED   e.g. Able to buy and/or prepare adequate meals independently. Online food shopping/takeaway food

1 = MET NEED   e.g. Unable to prepare food or drinks and has meals or assistance provided to meet need. Has foodbank vouchers

2 = UNMET NEED   e.g. Very restricted diet; culturally inappropriate food; unable to obtain adequate food; difficulty swallowing food. Needs foodbank vouchers

9 = NOT KNOWN

IF RATED 0 OR 9 GO TO QUESTION 5

HOW MUCH HELP DOES THE PERSON RECEIVE FROM RELATIVES OR FRIENDS WITH GETTING ENOUGH TO EAT?

0 = NONE

1 = LOW HELP   e.g. Occasional meal provided and/or occasional help with shopping/online orders.

2 = MODERATE HELP   e.g. Help with weekly shopping and/or meals provided more than weekly, but not daily.

3 = HIGH HELP   e.g. Assistance with food provided daily.

9 = NOT KNOWN

HOW MUCH HELP DOES THE PERSON RECEIVE FROM LOCAL SERVICES WITH GETTING ENOUGH TO EAT

HOW MUCH HELP DOES THE PERSON NEED FROM LOCAL SERVICES WITH GETTING ENOUGH TO EAT

0 = NONE

1 = LOW HELP   e.g. 1-4 meals a week provided or assisted for one meal a week.

2 = MODERATE HELP   e.g. More than 4 meals a week provided or assisted for all meals. Weekly shopping.

3 = HIGH HELP   e.g. All meals provided. Receives foodbank vouchers

9 = NOT KNOWN

DOES THE PERSON RECEIVE THE RIGHT TYPE OF HELP WITH GETTING ENOUGH TO EAT? (0 = NO   1 = YES   9 = NOT KNOWN)

OVERALL, IS THE PERSON SATISFIED WITH THE AMOUNT OF HELP THEY ARE RECEIVING WITH GETTING ENOUGH TO EAT?
(0 = NOT SATISFIED   1 = SATISFIED   9 = NOT KNOWN)

COMMENTS

4. SELF CARE

ASSESSMENTS
user   carer   staff   rater

DOES THE PERSON HAVE DIFFICULTY WITH SELF CARE?

Are you having any difficulty with personal care like washing, cutting your nails or dressing?
Do you ever need help?

0 = NO NEED   e.g. Appropriately dressed and groomed independently.

1 = MET NEED   e.g. Needs and gets appropriate help with self care.

2 = UNMET NEED   e.g. Poor personal hygiene, unable to wash or dress, not receiving appropriate help.

9 = NOT KNOWN

IF RATED 0 OR 9 GO TO QUESTION 5

HOW MUCH HELP DOES THE PERSON RECEIVE FROM RELATIVES OR FRIENDS WITH SELF CARE?

0 = NONE

1 = LOW HELP   e.g. Prompts (e.g. to change clothes) or helps occasionally.

2 = MODERATE HELP   e.g. Regular assistance e.g. weekly or more often.

3 = HIGH HELP   e.g. Daily assistance with care e.g. dressing, bathing: weekly laundry.

9 = NOT KNOWN

HOW MUCH HELP DOES THE PERSON RECEIVE FROM LOCAL SERVICES WITH SELF CARE?

HOW MUCH HELP DOES THE PERSON NEED FROM LOCAL SERVICES WITH SELF CARE?

0 = NONE

1 = LOW HELP   e.g.   Occasional prompting by staff.

2 = MODERATE HELP   e.g.   Supervise weekly washing and some other aspects of self-care

3 = HIGH HELP   e.g.   Supervise most aspects of self care: assist most days.

9 = NOT KNOWN

DOES THE PERSON RECEIVE THE RIGHT TYPE OF HELP WITH SELF CARE?   (0 = NO   1 = YES   9 = NOT KNOWN)

OVERALL, IS THE PERSON SATISFIED WITH THE AMOUNT OF HELP THEY ARE RECEIVING WITH SELF CARE?
(0 = NOT SATISFIED   1 = SATISFIED   9 = NOT KNOWN)

COMMENTS

5. CARING FOR SOMEONE ELSE

ASSESSMENTS
user   carer   staff   rater

DOES THE PERSON HAVE DIFFICULTY CARING FOR ANOTHER PERSON?

Is there anyone that you are caring for? Do you have any difficulty in looking after them?
Do you have childcare responsibilities (e.g. for grandchildren)?

0 = NO NEED   e.g. No-one to care for or no problem in caring.

1 = MET NEED   e.g. Difficulties with caring and receiving help.

2 = UNMET NEED   e.g. Serious difficulty in looking after or caring for another person.

9 = NOT KNOWN

IF RATED 0 OR 9 GO TO QUESTION 6

HOW MUCH HELP DOES THE PERSON RECEIVE FROM RELATIVES OR FRIENDS WITH LOOKING AFTER SOMEONE ELSE?

0 = NONE

1 = LOW HELP   e.g. Occasional help, less than once a week.

2 = MODERATE HELP   e.g. Help most days.

3 = HIGH HELP   e.g. Cared for person goes to stay with friends or relatives, assistance required everyday.

9 = NOT KNOWN

HOW MUCH HELP DOES THE PERSON RECEIVE FROM LOCAL SERVICES WITH CARING?

HOW MUCH HELP DOES THE PERSON NEED FROM LOCAL SERVICES WITH CARING?

0 = NONE

1 = LOW HELP   e.g. Person goes to day care: weekly assistance at home.

2 = MODERATE HELP   e.g. Nearly daily assistance at home, on-going carer support/training for user

3 = HIGH HELP   e.g. Respite care, 24-hour package or plans for alternative care for the cared for person.

9 = NOT KNOWN

DOES THE PERSON RECEIVE THE RIGHT TYPE OF HELP WITH CARING? (0 = NO   1 = YES   9 = NOT KNOWN)

OVERALL, IS THE PERSON SATISFIED WITH THE AMOUNT OF HELP THEY ARE RECEIVING WITH CARING?
(0 = NOT SATISFIED   1 = SATISFIED   9 = NOT KNOWN)

COMMENTS

6. DAYTIME ACTIVITIES

ASSESSMENTS
user   carer   staff   rater

DOES THE PERSON HAVE DIFFICULTY WITH REGULAR,
APPROPRIATE DAYTIME ACTIVITIES?

How do you spend your day? Do you have enough to do?

0 = NO NEED   e.g. Adequate social, work, leisure or learning activities, can arrange own activities.
                                    Computer literate – access to social media/internet

1 = MET NEED   e.g. Some limitation in occupying self, has appropriate activities organised by others.

2 = UNMET NEED   e.g. No adequate social, work or leisure activities.

9 = NOT KNOWN

IF RATED 0 OR 9 GO TO QUESTION 7

HOW MUCH HELP DOES THE PERSON RECEIVE FROM
RELATIVES OR FRIENDS IN FINDING OR KEEPING REGULAR
AND APPROPRIATE DAYTIME ACTIVITIES?

0 = NONE

1 = LOW HELP   e.g. Occasional help in arranging activities.

2 = MODERATE HELP   e.g. Help at least weekly.

3 = HIGH HELP   e.g. Daily help with arranging or providing activities.

9 = NOT KNOWN

HOW MUCH HELP DOES THE PERSON RECEIVE FROM LOCAL
SERVICES IN FINDING OR KEEPING REGULAR AND
APPROPRIATE ACTIVITIES?

HOW MUCH HELP DOES THE PERSON NEED FROM LOCAL
SERVICES IN FINDING OR KEEPING REGULAR AND
APPROPRIATE ACTIVITIES?

0 = NONE

1 = LOW HELP   e.g. Adult Education. Weekly day activity.

2 = MODERATE HELP   e.g. Day centre 2-4 days a week. Day Hospital attendance.
                                    Adequate activities 2-4 days week

3 = HIGH HELP   e.g. Provision of suitable activity 5 or more days per week e.g. day hospital or day centre

9 = NOT KNOWN

DOES THE PERSON RECEIVE THE RIGHT TYPE OF HELP WITH
ACTIVITIES? (0 = NO   1 = YES   9 = NOT KNOWN)

OVERALL, IS THE PERSON SATISFIED WITH THE AMOUNT OF
HELP THEY ARE RECEIVING WITH ACTIVITIES?
(0 = NOT SATISFIED   1 = SATISFIED   9 = NOT KNOWN)

COMMENTS

7. MEMORY

ASSESSMENTS

user   carer   staff   rater

DOES THE PERSON HAVE A PROBLEM WITH MEMORY?

Do you often have a problem remembering things that happened recently?
Do you often forget where you've put things?

0 = NO NEED   e.g. Occasionally forgets, but remembers later. No problem with memory.

1 = MET NEED   e.g. Some problems, but having investigations / assistance. Effective use of memory aids

2 = UNMET NEED   e.g. Clear deficit in recalling new information: loses things: becomes disorientated in time
                          and/or place, not receiving appropriate assistance. Needs diagnostic assessment

9 = NOT KNOWN

IF RATED 0 OR 9 GO TO QUESTION 8

HOW MUCH HELP DOES THE PERSON RECEIVE FROM RELATIVES OR FRIENDS FOR MEMORY LOSS?

0 = NONE

1 = LOW HELP   e.g. Prompting, occasional notes, reminders.

2 = MODERATE HELP   e.g. Assistance / supervision most days. Use of daily diary/calendar

3 = HIGH HELP   e.g. Living with relative. Constant supervision.

9 = NOT KNOWN

HOW MUCH HELP DOES THE PERSON RECEIVE FROM LOCAL SERVICES FOR MEMORY LOSS?

HOW MUCH HELP DOES THE PERSON NEED FROM LOCAL SERVICES FOR MEMORY LOSS?

0 = NONE

1 = LOW HELP   e.g. Some advice/ assistance with memory, GP clinic reviews.

2 = MODERATE HELP   e.g. Undergoing investigations. Regularly sees health care professional, e.g.
                          Memory Clinic, Day Hospital, Specialist day facility. Modified environment.

3 = HIGH HELP   e.g. Specially modified care because of memory needs. Intensive assistance.
                          Referral to memory clinic needed

9 = NOT KNOWN

DOES THE PERSON RECEIVE THE RIGHT TYPE OF HELP FOR MEMORY LOSS? (0 = NO   1 = YES   9 = NOT KNOWN)

OVERALL, IS THE PERSON SATISFIED WITH THE AMOUNT OF HELP THEY ARE RECEIVING FOR MEMORY LOSS?
(0 = NOT SATISFIED   1 = SATISFIED   9 = NOT KNOWN)

COMMENTS

8. EYESIGHT / HEARING /COMMUNICATION

ASSESSMENTS

user   carer   staff   rater

DOES THE PERSON HAVE A PROBLEM WITH SIGHT OR HEARING?

Do you have any difficulty hearing what someone says to you in a quiet room?
Do you have difficulty in seeing newsprint or watching television?
Are you able to express yourself clearly?

0 = NO NEED   e.g. No difficulties (wears appropriate corrective lenses or hearing aid, is independent).

1 = MET NEED   e.g. Some difficulty, but aids help to some extent, receiving appropriate investigations
                            or assistance to care for aids. Uses communication tools,

2 = UNMET NEED   e.g. A lot of difficulty seeing, hearing or expressing themselves, does not receive appropriate
                            assistance. Can sign signature

9 = NOT KNOWN

IF RATED 0 OR 9 GO TO QUESTION 9

HOW MUCH HELP DOES THE PERSON RECEIVE FROM RELATIVES OR FRIENDS WITH EYESIGHT/HEARING?

0 = NONE

1 = LOW HELP   e.g. Help making appointments for sight/ hearing problems. Occasional assistance

2 = MODERATE HELP   e.g. Regular help with difficult tasks e.g. reading correspondence.

3 = HIGH HELP   e.g. Help with most tasks that are difficult because of hearing/vision problem.

9 = NOT KNOWN

HOW MUCH HELP DOES THE PERSON RECEIVE FROM LOCAL SERVICES WITH EYESIGHT/ HEARING

HOW MUCH HELP DOES THE PERSON NEED FROM LOCAL SERVICES WITH EYESIGHT/ HEARING?

0 = NONE

1 = LOW HELP   e.g. Advice about impairment, aids provided or monitored. Prompts to use aids/glasses

2 = MODERATE HELP   e.g. Investigations/ treatment. Aids regularly formally reviewed. Regular assistance
                                with tasks.

3 = HIGH HELP   e.g. Assistance several days a week. Hospital appointments / specialist services or
                                specialist day facilities. Referral for eyesight/hearing problems needed

9 = NOT KNOWN

DOES THE PERSON RECEIVE THE RIGHT TYPE OF HELP WITH EYESIGHT / HEARING? (0 = NO   1 = YES   9 = NOT KNOWN)

OVERALL, IS THE PERSON SATISFIED WITH THE AMOUNT OF HELP THEY ARE RECEIVING WITH EYESIGHT/ HEARING?
(0 = NOT SATISFIED   1 = SATISFIED   9 = NOT KNOWN)

COMMENTS

9. MOBILITY / FALLS

ASSESSMENTS
user   carer   staff   rater

DOES THE PERSON HAVE RESTRICTED MOBILITY, FALLS OR ANY PROBLEMS USING PUBLIC TRANSPORT?

Do you have trouble moving about your home? Do you have falls or experience dizziness/loss of balance? Do you have trouble with transport?

0 = NO NEED	e.g. Physically able and mobile. Has mobility car allowance
1 = MET NEED	e.g. Some difficulty walking, climbing steps or using public transport, but able with assistance (e.g. walking aids, wheelchair). Occasional fall. Safety plan in place.
2 = UNMET NEED	e.g. Very restricted mobility even with walking aid. Frequent falls. Lack of appropriate help.
9 = NOT KNOWN	

IF RATED 0 OR 9 GO TO QUESTION 10

HOW MUCH HELP DOES THE PERSON RECEIVE FROM RELATIVES OR FRIENDS FOR MOBILITY PROBLEMS

0 = NONE	
1 = LOW HELP	e.g. Occasional help e.g. with transport, support.
2 = MODERATE HELP	e.g. Regular help with mobility/ public transport. Help organising home access alterations.
3 = HIGH HELP	e.g. Daily help and supervision with mobility/ transport.
9 = NOT KNOWN	

HOW MUCH HELP DOES THE PERSON RECEIVE FROM LOCAL SERVICES FOR MOBILITY PROBLEMS

HOW MUCH HELP DOES THE PERSON NEED FROM LOCAL SERVICES FOR MOBILITY PROBLEMS?

0 = NONE	
1 = LOW HELP	e.g. Advice, one or more aids. Referral for wheelchair
2 = MODERATE HELP	e.g. Currently undergoing investigations and/or O.T./ Physiotherapy assessments, regular transport, e.g. to day centre, light mobility assistance given. Application to mobility car scheme/mobility scooter, Disabled parking space, Disability badge
3 = HIGH HELP	e.g. Fully appropriate home alterations and aids. Substantial assistance most days. Care home because of mobility needs. Needs referral to physiotherapy/falls clinics
9 = NOT KNOWN	

DOES THE PERSON RECEIVE THE RIGHT TYPE OF HELP FOR MOBILITY PROBLEMS? (0 = NO   1 = YES   9 = NOT KNOWN)

OVERALL, IS THE PERSON SATISFIED WITH THE AMOUNT OF HELP THEY ARE RECEIVING FOR MOBILITY PROBLEMS
(0 = NOT SATISFIED   1 = SATISFIED   9 = NOT KNOWN)

COMMENTS

10. CONTINENCE

ASSESSMENTS
user carer staff rater

DOES THE PERSON HAVE INCONTINENCE?

Do you ever have accidents/ find yourself wet if you can't get to the toilet quickly?
(How much of a problem? Ever any soiling? Are you getting any help?)

0 = NO NEED   e.g. No incontinence. Independent in managing incontinence.

1 = MET NEED   e.g. Some incontinence. Receiving appropriate help/ investigations.

2 = UNMET NEED   e.g. Regularly wet or soiled. Deteriorating in continence needing assessment.

9 = NOT KNOWN

IF RATED 0 OR 9 GO TO QUESTION 11

HOW MUCH HELP DOES THE PERSON RECEIVE FROM RELATIVES OR FRIENDS FOR INCONTINENCE?

0 = NONE

1 = LOW HELP   e.g. Prompts to maintain continence. Orders continence aids online/from local pharmacy

2 = MODERATE HELP   e.g. Regularly assists with laundry, hygiene and use of aids.

3 = HIGH HELP   e.g. Full assistance with continence (laundry, hygiene, aids).

9 = NOT KNOWN

HOW MUCH HELP DOES THE PERSON RECEIVE FROM LOCAL SERVICES FOR INCONTINENCE?

HOW MUCH HELP DOES THE PERSON NEED FROM LOCAL SERVICES FOR INCONTINENCE?

0 = NONE

1 = LOW HELP   e.g. Prompts to maintain continence and provision of aids.

2 = MODERATE HELP   e.g. Investigations/ treatment. Regular help with laundry, hygiene and aids.

3 = HIGH HELP   e.g. Planned medical intervention (e.g. surgery). Constant care and assistance because of incontinence (e.g. in care home). Substantial continence programme in place.

9 = NOT KNOWN

DOES THE PERSON RECEIVE THE RIGHT TYPE OF HELP FOR INCONTINENCE? (0 = NO   1 = YES   9 = NOT KNOWN)

OVERALL, IS THE PERSON SATISFIED WITH THE AMOUNT OF HELP THEY ARE RECEIVING FOR INCONTINENCE?
(0 = NOT SATISFIED   1 = SATISFIED   9 = NOT KNOWN)

COMMENTS

11. PHYSICAL HEALTH

ASSESSMENTS

user   carer   staff   rater

DOES THE PERSON HAVE ANY PHYSICAL ILLNESS?

How well do you feel physically?
Are you getting any treatment from your doctor for physical problems?

0 = NO NEED	e.g. Physically well. Receiving no medical interventions.
1 = MET NEED	e.g. Physical ailment such as high blood pressure under control, receiving appropriate treatment / investigation. Reviews of physical conditions. Receiving palliative care
2 = UNMET NEED	e.g. Untreated serious physical ailment. Significant pain. Awaiting major surgery. Dehydration/Malnutrition Referral to palliative care team needed. Insomnia.
9 = NOT KNOWN	

IF RATED 0 OR 9 GO TO QUESTION 12

HOW MUCH HELP DOES THE PERSON RECEIVE FROM
RELATIVES OR FRIENDS FOR PHYSICAL HEALTH PROBLEMS?

0 = NONE	
1 = LOW HELP	e.g. Arranging appointments to see doctor.
2 = MODERATE HELP	e.g. Accompanied regularly to doctor / clinics.
3 = HIGH HELP	e.g. Daily help with condition arising out of physical health problems, e.g. living with a relative while convalescing or ill.
9 = NOT KNOWN	

HOW MUCH HELP DOES THE PERSON RECEIVE FROM LOCAL
SERVICES FOR PHYSICAL HEALTH PROBLEMS?

HOW MUCH HELP DOES THE PERSON NEED FROM LOCAL
SERVICES FOR PHYSICAL HEALTH PROBLEMS?

0 = NONE	
1 = LOW HELP	e.g. Given dietary or health advice. Occasional visit to GP for medicines.
2 = MODERATE HELP	e.g. Prescribed significant medications. Regularly seen by health care professional (GP, nurse, day hospital staff, outpatient clinic). Supplements provided
3 = HIGH HELP	e.g. Inpatient admissions, 24-hour nursing care. Very regular or intensive treatment.
9 = NOT KNOWN	

DOES THE PERSON RECEIVE THE RIGHT TYPE OF HELP FOR
PHYSICAL HEALTH PROBLEMS? (0 = NO   1 = YES   9 = NOT KNOWN)

OVERALL, IS THE PERSON SATISFIED WITH THE AMOUNT OF
HELP THEY ARE RECEIVING FOR PHYSICAL HEALTH
PROBLEMS? (0 = NOT SATISFIED   1 = SATISFIED   9 = NOT KNOWN)

COMMENTS

NB: consider oral health, skin care and foot care particularly in those people who are very frail or who have chronic medical conditions

12. DRUGS

DOES THE PERSON HAVE PROBLEMS WITH MEDICATION OR DRUGS?

Do you have any problems (e.g. side effects) with medication? How much medication are you on? Has your medication been recently reviewed by your doctor? Do you take any drugs that are not prescribed?

0 = NO NEED   e.g. No problems with compliance, side effects, drug abuse or dependency.

1 = MET NEED   e.g. Regular reviews, advice, District Nurse/ CPN administers medication, Dosette boxes/ aids

2 = UNMET NEED e.g. Poor compliance, dependency or abuse of prescribed or non-prescribed drugs. Inappropriate medication given. Use of illicit substances. Sharing of prescription. Hoarding of medication.

9 = NOT KNOWN

IF RATED 0 OR 9 GO TO QUESTION 13

HOW MUCH HELP DOES THE PERSON RECEIVE FROM RELATIVES OR FRIENDS WITH THEIR MEDICATION?

0 = NONE

1 = LOW HELP   e.g. Occasional prompt. Advice about drug misuse.

2 = MODERATE HELP e.g. Collection, regular reminding and checking of medication. Advice about agencies.

3 = HIGH HELP   e.g. Administers and holds medication. Support during drug withdrawal programme.

9 = NOT KNOWN

HOW MUCH HELP DOES THE PERSON RECEIVE FROM LOCAL SERVICES WITH THEIR MEDICATION?

HOW MUCH HELP DOES THE PERSON NEED FROM LOCAL SERVICES WITH THEIR MEDICATION?

0 = NONE

1 = LOW HELP   e.g. Advice from GP. Prompts to take medication.

2 = MODERATE HELP e.g. Supervision by District Nurse/ CPN/ Day Hospital/ care facility administers drugs.

3 = HIGH HELP   e.g. Intensive program regarding drug administration, compliance, abuse, or dependency (e.g., supervised withdrawal programme for drug dependency. Review of medication needed

9 = NOT KNOWN

DOES THE PERSON RECEIVE THE RIGHT TYPE OF HELP WITH MEDICATION? (0 = NO   1 = YES   9 = NOT KNOWN)

OVERALL, IS THE PERSON SATISFIED WITH THE AMOUNT OF HELP THEY ARE RECEIVING WITH THEIR MEDICATION?
(0 = NOT SATISFIED   1 = SATISFIED   9 = NOT KNOWN)

COMMENTS

13. PSYCHOTIC SYMPTOMS

DOES THE PERSON HAVE SYMPTOMS SUCH AS DELUSIONAL BELIEFS, HALLUCINATIONS, FORMAL THOUGHT DISORDER OR PASSIVITY?

Do you ever hear voices or see things that other people do not? Do you ever think that people are trying to harm you, or steal from you when they are not?
Are you on medication for this?

0 = NO NEED   e.g. No definite symptoms. Not at risk or in distress from symptoms and not on medication for psychotic symptoms.

1 = MET NEED   e.g. Symptoms helped by medication or other help e.g., coping strategies, safety plan.

2 = UNMET NEED   e.g. Currently has untreated symptoms or medication is not helping. Symptoms due to possible delirium. High levels of agitation

9 = NOT KNOWN

IF RATED 0 OR 9 GO TO QUESTION 14

HOW MUCH HELP DOES THE PERSON RECEIVE FROM RELATIVES OR FRIENDS FOR THESE PSYCHOTIC SYMPTOMS?

0 = NONE

1 = LOW HELP   e.g. Some support.

2 = MODERATE HELP   e.g. Carers involved in helping with coping strategies or medication compliance.

3 = HIGH HELP   e.g. Constant supervision of medication and helping with coping strategies.

9 = NOT KNOWN

HOW MUCH HELP DOES THE PERSON RECEIVE FROM LOCAL SERVICES FOR THESE PSYCHOTIC SYMPTOMS?

HOW MUCH HELP DOES THE PERSON NEED FROM LOCAL SERVICES FOR THESE PSYCHOTIC SYMPTOMS?

0 = NONE

1 = LOW HELP   e.g. Mental state and medication reviewed every three months or less often, support group.

2 = MODERATE HELP   e.g. Mental state and medication reviewed more frequently than every three months. Frequent specific therapy e.g. day hospital, high CPN input. Monthly depot.

3 = HIGH HELP   e.g. Active treatment/ 24-hour hospital care, daily day care or crisis care at home.

9 = NOT KNOWN

DOES THE PERSON RECEIVE THE RIGHT TYPE OF HELP FOR THESE SYMPTOMS? (0 = NO   1 = YES   9 = NOT KNOWN)

OVERALL, IS THE PERSON SATISFIED WITH THE AMOUNT OF HELP THEY ARE RECEIVING FOR THESE SYMPTOMS?
(0 = NOT SATISFIED   1 = SATISFIED   9 = NOT KNOWN)

COMMENTS

14. PSYCHOLOGICAL DISTRESS

ASSESSMENTS
user   carer   staff   rater

DOES THE PERSON SUFFER FROM CURRENT PSYCHOLOGICAL DISTRESS?

Have you recently felt very sad or fed up? Have you felt very anxious, frightened or worried?

0 = NO NEED   e.g. Occasional or mild distress. Copes independently

1 = MET NEED   e.g. Needs and gets on-going support.

2 = UNMET NEED   e.g. Distress affects life significantly, e.g. prevents person going out. Agitation

9 = NOT KNOWN

IF RATED 0 OR 9 GO TO QUESTION 15

HOW MUCH HELP DOES THE PERSON RECEIVE FROM RELATIVES OR FRIENDS FOR THIS DISTRESS?

0 = NONE

1 = LOW HELP   e.g. Some sympathy and support.

2 = MODERATE HELP   e.g. Has opportunity at least once a week to talk about distress and get help with
                                          coping strategies. Peer support provided. Access to online forums

3 = HIGH HELP   e.g. Constant support and supervision.

9 = NOT KNOWN

HOW MUCH HELP DOES THE PERSON RECEIVE FROM LOCAL SERVICES FOR THIS DISTRESS?

HOW MUCH HELP DOES THE PERSON NEED FROM LOCAL SERVICES FOR THIS DISTRESS?

0 = NONE

1 = LOW HELP   e.g. Assessment of mental state or occasional support.

2 = MODERATE HELP   e.g. Specific psychological or social intervention for distress. Counselled by staff at least
                                          once a week e.g. at Day Hospital. Access to telephone helpline

3 = HIGH HELP   e.g. 24-hour hospital care, or crisis care at home, daily assistance for distress.
                                          Needs referral for psychological support. Unresolved trauma

9 = NOT KNOWN

DOES THE PERSON RECEIVE THE RIGHT TYPE OF HELP FOR THIS DISTRESS? (0 = NO   1 = YES   9 = NOT KNOWN)

OVERALL, IS THE PERSON SATISFIED WITH THE AMOUNT OF HELP THEY ARE RECEIVING FOR THIS DISTRESS
(0 = NOT SATISFIED   1 = SATISFIED   9 = NOT KNOWN)

COMMENTS

15. INFORMATION (ON CONDITION & TREATMENT)

ASSESSMENTS
user   carer   staff   rater

HAS THE PERSON HAD CLEAR VERBAL OR WRITTEN
INFORMATION ABOUT THEIR CONDITION AND TREATMENT?

Have you been given clear information about your condition, medication or other treatment?
Do you want such information? How helpful has the information been?

0 = NO NEED   e.g. Has received and understood adequate information. Has not received but does
                              not want information.

1 = MET NEED   e.g. Receives assistance to understand information. Information given that is appropriate for
                              the person's level of communication / understanding.

2 = UNMET NEED   e.g. Has received inadequate or no information. Lack of mental capacity

9 = NOT KNOWN

IF RATED 0 OR 9 GO TO QUESTION 16

HOW MUCH HELP DOES THE PERSON RECEIVE FROM
RELATIVES OR FRIENDS IN OBTAINING SUCH INFORMATION?

0 = NONE

1 = LOW HELP   e.g. Some advice. Signposting to online internet sources.

2 = MODERATE HELP   e.g. Given leaflets/ fact-sheets or put in touch with self help groups.

3 = HIGH HELP   e.g. Regular liaison with mental health staff or voluntary groups (e.g. Alzheimer's
                                  Society) by friends or relatives. Lacks capacity, has nominated consultee.

9 = NOT KNOWN

HOW MUCH HELP DOES THE PERSON RECEIVE FROM LOCAL
SERVICES IN OBTAINING SUCH INFORMATION?

HOW MUCH HELP DOES THE PERSON NEED FROM LOCAL
SERVICES IN OBTAINING SUCH INFORMATION?

0 = NONE

1 = LOW HELP   e.g. Brief verbal or written information on illness/ problem/ treatment.

2 = MODERATE HELP   e.g. Given details of self-help groups. Long verbal information sessions e.g.
                                during Day Hospital attendance.

3 = HIGH HELP   e.g. Has been given specific personal education with or without detailed written information.
                                  Lacks capacity needs nominated consultee

9 = NOT KNOWN

DOES THE PERSON RECEIVE THE RIGHT TYPE OF HELP IN
OBTAINING INFORMATION?   (0 = NO   1 = YES   9 = NOT KNOWN)

OVERALL, IS THE PERSON SATISFIED WITH THE AMOUNT OF
HELP THEY ARE RECEIVING IN OBTAINING INFORMATION?
(0 = NOT SATISFIED   1 = SATISFIED   9 = NOT KNOWN)

COMMENTS

16. DELIBERATE SELF-HARM

ASSESSMENTS
user   carer   staff   rater

IS THE PERSON A DANGER TO THEMSELVES?

Do you ever think of harming yourself or actually tried to harm yourself?

0 = NO NEED   e.g. No thoughts of self-harm or suicide.

1 = MET NEED   e.g. Suicide risk monitored by staff, receiving counselling, adequate safety plan in place.

2 = UNMET NEED   e.g. Has expressed suicidal intent, deliberately neglected self or exposed self to serious danger in the last month. Self-harming behaviour

9 = NOT KNOWN

IF RATED 0 OR 9 GO TO QUESTION 17

HOW MUCH HELP DOES THE PERSON RECEIVE FROM RELATIVES OR FRIENDS TO REDUCE RISK OF DELIBERATE SELF HARM?

0 = NONE

1 = LOW HELP   e.g. Able to contact friends or relatives if feeling unsafe.

2 = MODERATE HELP   e.g. Friends or relatives are usually in contact and are likely to know if feeling unsafe.

3 = HIGH HELP   e.g. Friends or relatives in regular contact and are very likely to know and provide help if feeling unsafe.

9 = NOT KNOWN

HOW MUCH HELP DOES THE PERSON RECEIVE FROM LOCAL SERVICES TO REDUCE THE RISK OF DELIBERATE SELF-HARM?

HOW MUCH HELP DOES THE PERSON NEED FROM LOCAL SERVICES TO REDUCE THE RISK OF DELIBERATE SELF-HARM?

0 = NONE

1 = LOW HELP   e.g. Someone to contact if feeling unsafe.

2 = MODERATE HELP   e.g. Staff check at least once a week: regular supportive counselling.

3 = HIGH HELP   e.g. Daily supervision: inpatient care because of risk. Needs constant supervision

9 = NOT KNOWN

DOES THE PERSON RECEIVE THE RIGHT TYPE OF HELP TO REDUCE RISK OF DELIBERATE SELF-HARM?
(0 = NO   1 = YES   9 = NOT KNOWN)

OVERALL, IS THE PERSON SATISFIED WITH THE AMOUNT OF HELP THEY ARE RECEIVING TO REDUCE RISK OF DELIBERATE SELF-HARM? (0 = NOT SATISFIED   1 = SATISFIED   9 = NOT KNOWN)

COMMENTS

17. INADVERTENT SELF-HARM

ASSESSMENTS

user   carer   staff   rater

IS THE PERSON AT INADVERTENT RISK TO THEMSELVES?

Do you ever do anything that accidentally puts yourself in danger (e.g. leaving gas taps on, leaving fire unattended or getting lost)?

0 = NO NEED   e.g. No accidental self-harm.

1 = MET NEED   e.g. Specific supervision or help to prevent harm: e.g. memory notes, prompts, secure environment, observation. Use of assistive technology e.g. GPS tracker, Safekey

2 = UNMET NEED   e.g. Dangerous behaviour, e.g. getting lost, gas/ fire hazard, no appropriate safety plan. Risk assessment needed

9 = NOT KNOWN

IF RATED 0 OR 9 GO TO QUESTION 18

HOW MUCH HELP DOES THE PERSON RECEIVE FROM RELATIVES OR FRIENDS TO REDUCE RISK OF INADVERTENT SELF HARM

0 = NONE

1 = LOW HELP   e.g. Periodic supervision: weekly or less.

2 = MODERATE HELP   e.g. Supervision on 3-5 days a week.

3 = HIGH HELP   e.g. Almost constant supervision/ 24-hour care because of risk.

9 = NOT KNOWN

HOW MUCH HELP DOES THE PERSON RECEIVE FROM LOCAL SERVICES TO REDUCE THE RISK OF INADVERTENT SELF-HARM?

HOW MUCH HELP DOES THE PERSON NEED FROM LOCAL SERVICES TO REDUCE THE RISK OF INADVERTENT SELF-HARM?

0 = NONE

1 = LOW HELP   e.g. Check on behaviour weekly or less, risk assessment completed.

2 = MODERATE HELP   e.g. Daily Supervision, specific plan to prevent harm

3 = HIGH HELP   e.g. Constant supervision e.g. residential care because of risk for inadvertent self-harm.

9 = NOT KNOWN

DOES THE PERSON RECEIVE THE RIGHT TYPE OF HELP TO REDUCE RISK OF INADVERTENT SELF-HARM?
(0 = NO   1 = YES   9 = NOT KNOWN

OVERALL, IS THE PERSON SATISFIED WITH THE AMOUNT OF HELP THEY ARE RECEIVING TO REDUCE RISK OF HARM?
(0 = NOT SATISFIED   1 = SATISFIED   9 = NOT KNOWN)

COMMENTS

18. ABUSE/ NEGLECT

ASSESSMENTS
user   carer   staff   rater

IS THE PERSON AT RISK FROM OTHERS?

Has anyone done anything to frighten or harm you, or taken advantage of you?

0 = NO NEED   e.g. No abuse/ neglect issues over past month.

1 = MET NEED   e.g. Needs and gets ongoing support or protection. Safety plan in place. Use of caller screening.

2 = UNMET NEED   e.g. Regular shouting, pushing or neglect, financial misappropriation, physical assault. Vulnerable to exploitation. Safeguarding alert required

9 = NOT KNOWN

IF RATED 0 OR 9 GO TO QUESTION 19

HOW MUCH HELP DOES THE PERSON RECEIVE FROM RELATIVES OR FRIENDS TO REDUCE RISK OF ABUSE?

0 = NONE

1 = LOW HELP   e.g. Occasional advice.

2 = MODERATE HELP e.g. Regular support and protection.

3 = HIGH HELP   e.g. Constant support: very regular protection: negotiation.

9 = NOT KNOWN

HOW MUCH HELP DOES THE PERSON RECEIVE FROM LOCAL SERVICES TO REDUCE THE RISK OF ABUSE?

HOW MUCH HELP DOES THE PERSON NEED FROM LOCAL SERVICES TO REDUCE THE RISK OF ABUSE?

0 = NONE

1 = LOW HELP   e.g. Someone to contact when feeling threatened.

2 = MODERATE HELP e.g. Regular support: occasional respite.

3 = HIGH HELP   e.g. Constant supervision: legal involvement via services: separation from abuser. Safeguarding plan in place

9 = NOT KNOWN

DOES THE PERSON RECEIVE THE RIGHT TYPE OF HELP TO REDUCE RISK OF ABUSE? (0 = NO   1 = YES   9 = NOT KNOWN)

OVERALL, IS THE PERSON SATISFIED WITH THE AMOUNT OF HELP THEY ARE RECEIVING TO REDUCE RISK OF ABUSE?
(0 = NOT SATISFIED   1 = SATISFIED   9 = NOT KNOWN)

COMMENTS

19. BEHAVIOUR

IS THE PERSON'S BEHAVIOUR DANGEROUS, THREATENING, INTERFERING OR ANNOYING TO OTHERS?

Do you come into conflict with others e.g. by interfering with their affairs, frequently annoying, threatening or disturbing them? What happens?

0 = NO NEED   e.g. No history of disturbance to others.

1 = MET NEED   e.g. Under supervision / treatment because of potential risk.

2 = UNMET NEED   e.g. Recent violence, threats or seriously interfering behaviour. High levels of agitation

9 = NOT KNOWN

IF RATED 0 OR 9 GO TO QUESTION 20

HOW MUCH HELP DOES THE PERSON RECEIVE FROM RELATIVES OR FRIENDS TO REDUCE ANNOYING OR DISTURBING BEHAVIOUR?

0 = NONE

1 = LOW HELP   e.g. Help/ supervision weekly or less.

2 = MODERATE HELP   e.g. Help/ supervision more often than weekly.

3 = HIGH HELP   e.g. Almost constant help/ supervision due to persistently disturbing behaviour.

9 = NOT KNOWN

HOW MUCH HELP DOES THE PERSON RECEIVE FROM LOCAL SERVICES TO REDUCE ANNOYING OR DISTURBING BEHAVIOUR?

HOW MUCH HELP DOES THE PERSON NEED FROM LOCAL SERVICES TO REDUCE ANNOYING OR DISTURBING BEHAVIOUR?

0 = NONE

1 = LOW HELP   e.g. Check on behaviour weekly or less.

2 = MODERATE HELP   e.g. Daily supervision or night-sitting service, active care plan in place.

3 = HIGH HELP   e.g. Constant supervision: intensive behaviour management programme.

9 = NOT KNOWN

DOES THE PERSON RECEIVE THE RIGHT TYPE OF HELP TO REDUCE ANNOYING OR DISTURBING BEHAVIOUR?
(0 = NO   1 = YES   9 = NOT KNOWN)

OVERALL, IS THE PERSON SATISFIED WITH THE AMOUNT OF HELP THEY ARE RECEIVING TO REDUCE DISTURBING BEHAVIOUR? (0 = NOT SATISFIED   1 = SATISFIED   9 = NOT KNOWN)

COMMENTS

20. ALCOHOL

ASSESSMENTS

user   carer   staff   rater

DOES THE PERSON DRINK EXCESSIVELY OR HAVE A PROBLEM CONTROLLING THEIR DRINKING?

Do you drink alcohol? How much? Does drinking cause you any problems?
Do you ever feel guilty about it? Do you ever wish you could cut down your drinking?

0 = NO NEED   e.g. Doesn't drink or drinks sensibly.

1 = MET NEED   e.g. At risk from alcohol abuse and receiving assistance.

2 = UNMET NEED   e.g. Current drinking harmful or uncontrollable, not receiving appropriate assistance.

9 = NOT KNOWN

IF RATED 0 OR 9 GO TO QUESTION 21

HOW MUCH HELP DOES THE PERSON RECEIVE FROM RELATIVES OR FRIENDS FOR THEIR DRINKING?

0 = NONE

1 = LOW HELP   e.g. Advised to cut down.

2 = MODERATE HELP e.g. Advised about helping agencies, e.g. Alcoholics Anonymous.

3 = HIGH HELP   e.g. Constant support and/ or monitoring of alcohol intake.

9 = NOT KNOWN

HOW MUCH HELP DOES THE PERSON RECEIVE FROM LOCAL SERVICES FOR THEIR DRINKING?

HOW MUCH HELP DOES THE PERSON NEED FROM LOCAL SERVICES FOR THEIR DRINKING?

0 = NONE

1 = LOW HELP   e.g. Given information and told about risks.

2 = MODERATE HELP e.g. Given support and details of helping agencies, access to drink is supervised.

3 = HIGH HELP   e.g. Attends alcohol clinic, supervised withdrawal programme.

9 = NOT KNOWN

DOES THE PERSON RECEIVE THE RIGHT TYPE OF HELP FOR THEIR DRINKING? (0 = NO   1 = YES   9 = NOT KNOWN)

OVERALL, IS THE PERSON SATISFIED WITH THE AMOUNT OF HELP THEY ARE RECEIVING FOR THEIR DRINKING?
(0 = NOT SATISFIED   1 = SATISFIED   9 = NOT KNOWN)

COMMENTS

21. COMPANY

DOES THE PERSON NEED HELP WITH SOCIAL CONTACT?

Are you happy with your social life? Do you wish you had more social contact with others?

0 = NO NEED   e.g. Able to organise enough social contact, has enough contact with friends· Use of social media.

1 = MET NEED   e.g. Lack of company identified as a problem. Has specific intervention for company needs e.g., lonely at night but attends drop-in or day centre or Lunch Club. Social work involvement.

2 = UNMET NEED   e.g. Frequently feels lonely and isolated. Very few social contacts.

9 = NOT KNOWN

IF RATED 0 OR 9 GO TO QUESTION 22

HOW MUCH HELP DOES THE PERSON RECEIVE FROM RELATIVES OR FRIENDS WITH SOCIAL CONTACT?

0 = NONE

1 = LOW HELP   e.g. Friends help with social contact or visit less than weekly to provide company. Family or friends contact person on social media.

2 = MODERATE HELP   e.g. Friends help with social contact weekly or more often. Member of online internet groups.

3 = HIGH HELP   e.g. Friends help with social contact at least four times a week. Regular or daily contact on social media

9 = NOT KNOWN

HOW MUCH HELP DOES THE PERSON RECEIVE FROM LOCAL SERVICES IN ORGANISING SOCIAL CONTACT?

HOW MUCH HELP DOES THE PERSON NEED FROM LOCAL SERVICES IN ORGANISING SOCIAL CONTACT?

0 = NONE

1 = LOW HELP   e.g. Occasional visits from befriender or voluntary worker. Referral to centre.

2 = MODERATE HELP   e.g. Regular attendance at day centre: regular luncheon club, organised social activity.

3 = HIGH HELP   e.g. Day centre or social home visits 3 or more times a week, social skills training, social worker involvement.

9 = NOT KNOWN

DOES THE PERSON RECEIVE THE RIGHT TYPE OF HELP WITH SOCIAL CONTACT? (0 = NO   1 = YES   9 = NOT KNOWN)

OVERALL, IS THE PERSON SATISFIED WITH THE AMOUNT OF HELP THEY ARE RECEIVING WITH THEIR SOCIAL CONTACT?
(0 = NOT SATISFIED   1 = SATISFIED   9 = NOT KNOWN)

COMMENTS

22. INTIMATE RELATIONSHIPS

ASSESSMENTS
user   carer   staff   rater

DOES THE PERSON HAVE A PARTNER, RELATIVE OR FRIEND WITH WHOM THEY HAVE A CLOSE EMOTIONAL/ PHYSICAL RELATIONSHIP?

Do you have a partner, relative or friend you feel close to? Do you get on well?
Can you talk about your worries or problems? Do you lack physical contact/ intimacy?

0 = NO NEED	e.g. Happy with current relationships or does not want any intimate relationship.
1 = MET NEED	e.g. Has problems concerning intimate relationships, specific plan, counselling/ advice/ support which is helpful. Internet dating/online friendships
2 = UNMET NEED	e.g. Socially isolated lonely. Lack of close confidant or trusting relationship.
9 = NOT KNOWN	

IF RATED 0 OR 9 GO TO QUESTION 23

HOW MUCH HELP DOES THE PERSON RECEIVE FROM RELATIVES OR FRIENDS WITH INTIMATE RELATIONSHIPS OR LONELINESS?

0 = NONE	
1 = LOW HELP	e.g. Occasional emotional support.
2 = MODERATE HELP	e.g. Regular support.
3 = HIGH HELP	e.g. Help contacting counselling services (e.g. bereavement/ marriage counselling) and possibly accompanying the person there.
9 = NOT KNOWN	

HOW MUCH HELP DOES THE PERSON RECEIVE FROM LOCAL SERVICES WITH INTIMATE RELATIONSHIPS OR LONELINESS?

HOW MUCH HELP DOES THE PERSON NEED FROM LOCAL SERVICES WITH INTIMATE RELATIONSHIPS OR LONELINESS?

0 = NONE	
1 = LOW HELP	e.g. Some support/ advice
2 = MODERATE HELP	e.g. Regular support/ advice /contact.
3 = HIGH HELP	e.g. Intensive support. Specific therapy, e.g. marital or bereavement counselling.
9 = NOT KNOWN	

DOES THE PERSON RECEIVE THE RIGHT TYPE OF HELP WITH RELATIONSHIPS? (0 = NO   1 = YES   9 = NOT KNOWN)

OVERALL, IS THE PERSON SATISFIED WITH THE AMOUNT OF HELP THEY ARE RECEIVING WITH RELATIONSHIPS?
(0 = NOT SATISFIED   1 = SATISFIED   9 = NOT KNOWN)

COMMENTS

23. MONEY / BUDGETING

ASSESSMENTS
user   carer   staff   rater

DOES THE PERSON HAVE PROBLEMS MANAGING OR
BUDGETING THEIR MONEY?

Do you have any difficulty managing your money? Are you able to pay your bills?

0 = NO NEED   e.g. Able to buy essential items and pay bills independently. Use of online banking and utility
                              accounts. Use of credit card

1 = MET NEED   e.g. Benefits from help with managing affairs or budgeting. Shared access to online bank and
                              utility accounts.

2 = UNMET NEED e.g. Often has no money for essential items or bills. Unable to manage finances. Lasting
                              power of attorney needed. Needs debt repayment plan.

9 = NOT KNOWN

IF RATED 0 OR 9 GO TO QUESTION 24

HOW MUCH HELP DOES THE PERSON RECEIVE FROM
RELATIVES OR FRIENDS IN MANAGING THEIR MONEY?

0 = NONE

1 = LOW HELP   e.g. Occasional help sorting out household bills. Shared access to online bank and utility
                              accounts.

2 = MODERATE HELP e.g. Frequent assistance, calculating weekly budget, collecting pension. Shared credit
                              card

3 = HIGH HELP   e.g. Complete management of finances. Power of Attorney.

9 = NOT KNOWN

HOW MUCH HELP DOES THE PERSON RECEIVE FROM LOCAL
SERVICES IN MANAGING THEIR MONEY?

HOW MUCH HELP DOES THE PERSON NEED FROM LOCAL
SERVICES IN MANAGING THEIR MONEY?

0 = NONE

1 = LOW HELP   e.g. Occasional help with budgeting

2 = MODERATE HELP e.g. Supervised in paying rent, given weekly spending money

3 = HIGH HELP   e.g. Virtual or complete management of finances: Court of protection:
                              Lasting Power of Attorney

9 = NOT KNOWN

DOES THE PERSON RECEIVE THE RIGHT TYPE OF HELP IN
MANAGING THEIR MONEY? (0 = NO   1 = YES   9 = NOT KNOWN)

OVERALL, IS THE PERSON SATISFIED WITH THE AMOUNT OF
HELP THEY ARE RECEIVING IN MANAGING THEIR MONEY?
(0 = NOT SATISFIED   1 = SATISFIED   9 = NOT KNOWN)

COMMENTS

24. BENEFITS

ASSESSMENTS

user   carer   staff   rater

IS THE PERSON DEFINITELY RECEIVING ALL THE BENEFITS THAT THEY ARE ENTITLED TO?

Are you sure that you are getting all the money that you are entitled to?

0 = NO NEED   e.g. Has no need of benefits or receiving full entitlement of benefits.

1 = MET NEED   e.g. Receives appropriate help in claiming benefits, social worker involvement over past month.

2 = UNMET NEED   e.g. Not sure/ not receiving full entitlement of benefits. Needs welfare benefit check.
Emergency payment needed

9 = NOT KNOWN

IF RATED 0 OR 9 GO TO CARER'S SECTION OVERLEAF

HOW MUCH HELP DOES THE PERSON RECEIVE FROM RELATIVES OR FRIENDS IN OBTAINING THEIR FULL BENEFIT ENTITLEMENT?

0 = NONE

1 = LOW HELP   e.g. Occasionally asks whether person is getting any money.

2 = MODERATE HELP e.g. Make enquiries about entitlements and help fill in forms.

3 = HIGH HELP   e.g. Has ensured full benefits are being received.

9 = NOT KNOWN

HOW MUCH HELP DOES THE PERSON RECEIVE FROM LOCAL SERVICES IN OBTAINING THEIR FULL BENEFIT ENTITLEMENT?

HOW MUCH HELP DOES THE PERSON NEED FROM LOCAL SERVICES IN OBTAINING THEIR FULL BENEFIT ENTITLEMENT?

0 = NONE

1 = LOW HELP   e.g. Occasional advice about entitlements.

2 = MODERATE HELP e.g. Help with applying for extra entitlements.

3 = HIGH HELP   e.g. Comprehensive evaluation of current entitlement in past month.
Emergency payment needed.

9 = NOT KNOWN

DOES THE PERSON RECEIVE THE RIGHT TYPE OF HELP IN OBTAINING THEIR FULL BENEFIT ENTITLEMENT?
(0 = NO   1 = YES   9 = NOT KNOWN)

OVERALL, IS THE PERSON SATISFIED WITH THE AMOUNT OF HELP THEY ARE RECEIVING IN OBTAINING THEIR FULL BENEFIT ENTITLEMENT? (0 = NOT SATISFIED   1 = SATISFIED   9 = NOT KNOWN)

COMMENTS

A. CARERS NEED FOR INFORMATION

ASSESSMENTS
user   carer   staff   rater

HAS THE CARER BEEN GIVEN CLEAR INFORMATION ABOUT THE PERSONS CONDITION AND ALL THE TREATMENT AVAILABLE?

Have you been given clear information about X's condition and all the treatment and services available? How helpful has this information been?

0 = NO NEED   e.g. Received and understood. Aware of online resources.

1 = MET NEED   e.g. Has not received or understood all information, receives help with information.

2 = UNMET NEED   e.g. Has received little or no information, has not understood information given. Signposting to information needed. Needs referral to carer education group.

9 = NOT KNOWN

IF RATED 0 OR 9 GO TO QUESTION B

HOW MUCH HELP DOES THE CARER RECEIVE FROM RELATIVES OR FRIENDS IN OBTAINING SUCH INFORMATION?

0 = NONE

1 = LOW HELP   e.g. Has had some advice.

2 = MODERATE HELP   e.g. Given leaflets/ fact sheets or put in touch with self-help groups.

3 = HIGH HELP   e.g. Regular liaison with doctors, other professionals, self help or support groups by friends or relatives.

9 = NOT KNOWN

HOW MUCH HELP DOES THE CARER RECEIVE FROM LOCAL SERVICES IN OBTAINING SUCH INFORMATION?

HOW MUCH HELP DOES THE CARER NEED FROM LOCAL SERVICES IN OBTAINING SUCH INFORMATION?

0 = NONE

1 = LOW HELP   e.g. Brief verbal or written information on condition/ problem/ treatment.

2 = MODERATE HELP   e.g. Given details of self-help groups. Personal explanations of drugs, alternative treatments/ services and likely course of the condition. Signposting to online information resources and helplines

3 = HIGH HELP   e.g. Has been given detailed written information or has had specific personal education: e.g. from key worker.

9 = NOT KNOWN

DOES THE CARER RECEIVE THE RIGHT TYPE OF HELP IN OBTAINING SUCH INFORMATION? (0 = NO   1 = YES   9 = NOT KNOWN)

OVERALL, IS THE CARER SATISFIED WITH THE AMOUNT OF HELP THEY ARE RECEIVING IN OBTAINING SUCH INFORMATION? (0 = NOT SATISFIED   1 = SATISFIED   9 = NOT KNOWN)

COMMENTS

133

B. CARERS PSYCHOLOGICAL DISTRESS

ASSESSMENTS
user   carer   staff   rater

IS THE CARER CURRENTLY PSYCHOLOGICALLY DISTRESSED?

Do you find it difficult or stressful caring for X? Do you feel you need a break or much more support for yourself?

0 = NO NEED   e.g. Coping well.

1 = MET NEED   e.g. Some stress: receiving help/ contact/ support that is beneficial.

2 = UNMET NEED   e.g. Very stressed or depressed. Wants relief from caring. Family needs specialist nurse or carers worker involvement.

9 = NOT KNOWN

IF RATED 0 OR 9 FINISH

HOW MUCH HELP DOES THE CARER RECEIVE FROM RELATIVES OR FRIENDS FOR THIS DISTRESS?

0 = NONE

1 = LOW HELP   e.g. Occasional advice/ support.

2 = MODERATE HELP   e.g. Weekly practical and/ or emotional support and/ or relief from caring.

3 = HIGH HELP   e.g. Regular respite and assistance with tasks (e.g. 3-4 times per week).

9 = NOT KNOWN

HOW MUCH HELP DOES THE CARER RECEIVE FROM LOCAL SERVICES FOR THIS DISTRESS?

HOW MUCH HELP DOES THE CARER NEED FROM LOCAL SERVICES FOR THIS DISTRESS?

0 = NONE

1 = LOW HELP   e.g. Advice e.g. about other options such as residential care.

2 = MODERATE HELP e.g. Weekly day care: occasional respite: CPN visits: carers support groups. Dementia Advisor

3 = HIGH HELP   e.g. Regular respite admissions. Treatment and/ or counselling for stress/depression. Specialist nurse or carer worker involved

9 = NOT KNOWN

DOES THE CARER RECEIVE THE RIGHT TYPE OF HELP FOR THIS DISTRESS? (0 = NO   1 = YES   9 = NOT KNOWN)

OVERALL, IS THE CARER SATISFIED WITH THE AMOUNT OF HELP THEY ARE RECEIVING FOR THIS DISTRESS?
(0 = NOT SATISFIED   1 = SATISFIED   9 = NOT KNOWN)

COMMENTS

CANE Summary Sheet

User Name: _____   Date: _____

(Section 2-4b rater's overall ratings)

Section of the CANE	Section 1 Need				Section 2 Informal help	Section 3a Formal help	Section 3b Help needed	Section 4a Type of help	4b User Satisfaction
	U	C	S	R					
1. Accommodation									
2. Looking after the home									
3. Food									
4. Self Care									
5. Caring for someone else									
6. Daytime activities									
7. Memory									
8. Eyesight / Hearing									
9. Mobility / Falls									
10. Continence									
11. Physical Health									
12. Drugs									
13. Psychotic symptoms									
14. Psychological distress									
15. Information									
16. Safety to self									
17. Inadvertent self harm									
18. Abuse / Neglect									
19. Behaviour									
20. Alcohol									
21. Company									
22. Intimate relationships									
23. Money/Budgeting									
24. Benefits									
A. Carers need for information									
B. Carers psychological distress									
Met needs: Number of 1s in the column									
Unmet Needs: Number of 2s in the column									
Total Needs: Add number of Met needs and Unmet needs									
Total level of help given, needed, and satisfaction. (Add scores, rate 9 as 0)									

CAMBERWELL ASSESSMENT OF NEED FOR THE ELDERLY

(SHORT CANE)

Version I

CODE	

Interviewee	Date	Interview Time
User		
Staff		
Carer		
Rater/Clinician		

Background Details
(please fill in blanks, or circle whichever applies)

CODE NUMBER: _____

Date of Birth: _____ AGE: _____(years)

SEX: male / female

ETHNICITY: Asian/ African/ African-American/ Black Caribbean / White/ Other_____

RELIGION: Christian/Muslim/Hindu/Jewish/Other _____

FIRST LANGUAGE : English/Other _____

MARITAL STATUS: single / married / divorced / separated / widowed

LIVING SITUATION: alone / with partner / with other relatives / with others

LIVING ENVIRONMENT: flat / house / sheltered / residential / nursing / other

PREVIOUS OCCUPATION (or partner's): _____

EDUCATION: _____(years)

CURRENT STATUS: in-patient / day-patient / community patient (Psychiatric / Geriatric/other)

MAIN DIAGNOSES (DSM-IV/ICD 10): _____

_____

_____

_____

CURRENT MEDICATION: _____

_____

DISEASE PREVENTION: (e.g. blood pressure/smoking/sleep pattern/exercise/health screening/vaccination)

_____

DOES THE PERSON HAVE A CARER? yes / no
IS THE PERSON A CARER? yes / no

NOTES:

Instructions for the Short CANE

The Short CANE is a comprehensive, person-centred needs assessment tool that has been designed for use with the elderly. It is suitable for use in a variety of clinical and research settings. The CANE has a person-centred approach which allows views of the professional, user and carer to be recorded and compared. The instrument uses the principle that identifying a need means identifying a problem plus an appropriate intervention which will help or alleviate the need. Therefore, the CANE models clinical practice and relies on professional expertise for ratings to be completed accurately. Administrators need to have an adequate knowledge of clinical interviewing and decision-making. Administrators should also have good working knowledge of the concepts of need, met need and unmet need. This knowledge can be gained with experience of full CANE assessments and reference to the manual.

There are 24 topics relating to the user and two (A and B) relating to the carer. There are four columns to document ratings so that one or more of the user (U), staff member (S), carer (C) or rater (clinician/researcher) (R) can each express their view. Note at the top of the column which person has been interviewed.

The Short CANE aims to assess whether there is currently a need in the specific area. A *need* is defined as a problem with a potential remedy or intervention. Use the prompts below each area on the record form to establish the user's current status with regards to the need area. If there has been a need, then assess whether it was met appropriately. Score each interviewee independently, even though the user's perceptions of need in each area may differ from others. The administrator should ask additional questions probing into the area until he or she can establish whether the person has a significant need that requires assistance and whether he or she is getting enough of the right type of help. Once this information has been gathered, a rating of need can be made. Judgement of rating in this section should be based on normal clinical practice. The CANE is intended to be a framework for assessment grounded in good professional practice and expertise. Although Section 1 in each problem area is the main section of interest to CANE administrators, it often cannot be rated until adequate information has been collected about the area. When adequate information has been

gathered, the rater should clearly be able to make a clinical judgement as to whether the area is a met need, an unmet need or is not a need for the person. Confusion with ratings can be avoided by not directly asking a closed question about whether there is a problem in a certain area (e.g., 'Do you have any problems with the food here?') because the person can answer 'No'. This response may then be mistaken as a 'No need' where in fact it is a 'Met need' because the person is assisted by someone else.

♦ *No need:* Score 0 there if there is no need in the area; then go on to the next page. In this situation, the user is coping well independently and does not need any further assistance, for example, the user has reported that they are successfully administering their own medication and do not have any problematic side effects, or a staff member reports that the user appeared to be comfortable in his or her home environment and that no alterations to the building are needed or planned.

♦ *Met need:* Score 1 if the need is met or if there is a minor need requiring no significant intervention. A need is met when there is a mild, moderate or serious problem which is receiving an intervention that is appropriate and potentially of benefit. This category is also used for problems which would normally not be of clinical significance and would not require a specific intervention, for example, the user is receiving an assessment for poor eyesight or a district nurse is overseeing the administration of medications each day.

♦ *Unmet need:* Score 2 if the need is currently unmet. An unmet need is a serious problem requiring intervention or assessment, which is currently receiving no assistance or the *wrong* type or level of help, for example, if a staff member reported that the user was incontinent of large amounts of urine every night despite toileting twice during the night and the use of pads, or a carer reported that the user had become very hard of hearing and had not received an assessment or suitable hearing aids.

♦ *Unknown:* Score 9 if the person does not know about the nature of the problems or about the assistance the person receives; then go on to the next page. Such a score may mean that further information is needed to make a rating

Scoring

It is to be noted that scoring is a secondary aspect of the CANE, as its primary purpose is to identify and assess individual unmet needs. The total CANE score is based on the rating of Section 1 of each of the 24 problem areas. The two areas (A and B) relating to carer's needs are not added into this total score. Count the total number of met needs (rated as a 1 in Section 1) out of a maximum of 24. Count the total number of unmet needs identified (rated as a 2 in Section 1) out of a maximum of 24. Count the total number of needs identified (rated as a 1 or 2 in Section 1) out of a maximum of 24. The raters' (clinicians or researchers) ratings are made based on all the information gathered through the assessment. Raters' ratings of Section 1 are used as the basis for total CANE scores.

Short CANE

User Name: _____ Date: _____

Ratings: 0 = no need 1 = met need 2 = unmet need 9 = unknown

Interviewee: U = User C = Carer S = Staff R = researcher	U	C	S	R
1. ACCOMMODATION Does the person have an appropriate place to live?				
2. LOOKING AFTER THE HOME Is the person able to look after their home?				
3. FOOD Does the person get enough of the right type of food to eat?				
4. SELF CARE How does the person look after their self-care?				
5. CARING FOR SOMEONE ELSE Does the person care for another? Can they manage this caring?				
6. DAYTIME ACTIVITIES How does the person occupy their day?				
7. MEMORY Does the person have a problem with memory?				
8. EYESIGHT / HEARING How is the person's eyesight and hearing?				
9. MOBILITY / FALLS How does the person get around inside and outside their home?				
10. CONTINENCE Is the person continent?				
11. PHYSICAL HEALTH How is the person's physical health?				
12. DRUGS Does the person have problems with medication or drugs?				
13. PSYCHOTIC SYMPTOMS Does the person ever hear or see things other do not?				
14. PSYCHOLOGICAL DISTRESS Does the person have problems with mood or anxiety?				
15. INFORMATION (ON CONDITION & TREATMENT) Has the person had clear information about their condition?				
16. SAFETY TO SELF (DELIBERATE SELF-HARM) Is the person a danger to themselves?				
17. SAFETY TO SELF (INADVERTENT SELF-HARM) Does the person have accidents?				
18. SAFETY TO SELF (ABUSE/ NEGLECT) Is the person at risk from others?				
19. BEHAVIOUR Is the person's behaviour problematic for others?				
20. ALCOHOL Does the person have a drinking problem?				
21. COMPANY Does the person have an adequate social life?				
22. INTIMATE RELATIONSHIPS Does the person have a close emotional/physical relationship?				
23. MONEY/ BUDGETING How does the person manage their money?				
24. BENEFITS Is the person receiving the benefits he/she is entitled too?				
A. CARERS NEED FOR INFORMATION Has the carer been given all the information they need about the person's condition and treatment?				
B. CARERS PSYCHOLOGICAL DISTRESS Is the carer currently psychologically distressed?				
Met Needs: Count the number of 1s in the column (1 to 24 only).				
Unmet Needs: Count the number of 2s in the column (1 to 24 only)				
Total Needs: Add number of Met needs and Unmet needs (1 to 24 only)				

Index

abuse/neglect, 4, 38, 69
accommodation needs, 4, 20, 24, 28
activities of daily living (ADLs), 15,
    35–6, *see also* daytime activities
    needs
advance care planning, 15, 16
age as risk factor
    for long-term care, 87
    for people with depression in
        residential homes, 38
    for primary care patients, 21
ageing, demographic trends toward
    and dementia, 10
    in Korea, 52
    in Poland, 86
    in UK, 44
    in US, 44
    worldwide, 1, 44
alcohol needs, 25, 59, 83
Alzheimer's disease, 53, 77
Andersen model, 91, 92, 93
anosognosia, 29
anxiety, 15, 62, 88
Australia, 6, 77, 78

behavioural and psychological
    symptoms in dementia (BPSD), 17
benefits needs, 54, 59
bipolar disorder, 6
Brazil, 3

Camberwell Assessment of Need, 2
Camberwell Assessment of Need for
    the Elderly (CANE)
    adaptations of, 3–5
    amendments to, 100
    electronic version of, 100
    instructions for long version, 105–8
    instructions for short version, 138–9
    international use of, 3
    overview, 2
    structure of, 2
    time required to administer, 3, 99
    translations of, 3–4
Canada, 5
CANE. *see* Camberwell Assessment of
    Need for the Elderly (CANE)
cardiovascular diseases, 20, 21, 24–5,
    28

caregiver burden, 99
    alleviated by case management, 64
    of carers of people with dementia,
        52, 56–9
carers
    assessment of their relatives' needs,
        25, 28
    caregiver burden, 56–9
    causes of crises for, 62–3
    future research on, 99
    long-distance carers, 44, 49
    need for outside help, 56, 59
    of people with dementia, 10, 52, 64
    spouses and children of people with
        young-onset dementia, 80–2
caring for someone else (CANE
    category), 20, 54
case management, 14, 16, 63–4
Chile, 3
China, 4
chronic pain, 29
Cogknow Day Navigator, 98
communication. *see* eyesight/hearing/
    communication needs
community health, 5–6
community services
    and case management, 64
    needed by people with dementia and
        their carers, 56
company needs
    impact on caregiver burden, 59
    of people with dementia, 46, 54, 88
    of people with dementia living at
        home, 15, 16
    of people with depression, 6, 38, 39
    of people living alone, 48
    of people in long-term care, 87
    of people in residential homes,
        38
    of people in rural communities, 4
    of primary care patients, 20, 21, 26,
        27
continence needs, 24, 27, 79
continuity of care, 15, 16
coordination of health services,
    14, 16
costs of health care, 91–5
crises
    causes of, 62–3

interventions to prevent and
    manage, 63–5, 66–8, 72–3
    management of, 63
crisis intervention models, 63

daytime activities needs
    impact on caregiver burden, 56, 59
    of people with dementia, 46, 54
    of people with dementia living at
        home, 15, 17, 59
    of people with depression, 6,
        38, 40
    of people living alone, 46, 48
    of people in long-term care, 87–8
    of people in rural communities, 4
    of primary care patients, 20, 21, 25,
        26, 27
Delphi process, 65
DelpHi Standard, 11, 14
dementia, 6, 14, *see also* interventions
        for people with dementia
    caregiver burden of family carers,
        56–9
    crises, 62–3
    diagnosis and evaluation, 14,
        16, 78
    and environmental needs, 14–15, 16
    health outcomes in home
        environment, 62
    and people with depression in
        residential homes, 10–17, 40,
        45–9, 54–6, 88
    and primary care patients, 20–1, 24,
        29
    satisfaction with help received, 56,
        59
    and self-assessment of needs, 10
    statistics in the UK, 62
    symptoms, 10, 16, 78
    and technology use, 98–9
    young-onset, 77–84
depression, 6, 24–5
    and primary care patients, 20–1,
        24–6, 28–9
    difficulty of recognising in old age,
        28
    impact on self-reported needs, 6, 40
    and people in residential homes, 34,
        38–41, 87, 88

diagnosis
  of dementia, 14, 16
  of young-onset dementia, 78
disease awareness, 79, 80, 83

EASY-Care, 5
eyesight/hearing/communication
    needs
  of people with dementia living at
    home, 15–16, 46, 59
  of people with depression, 6, 38
  of people in long-term care, 87–8
  of people in residential homes, 38
  of primary care patients, 20, 24, 25,
    27, 28

falls. *see* mobility/falls needs
family carers. *see* carers
FIMA. *see* Questionnaire for Health-
    Related Resource Use in an
    Elderly Population (FIMA)
food needs. *see* nutritional needs

gender as risk factor, 38, 46, 87
general practitioners (GPs), 20
  and depression in older people,
    29
  inappropriate attitudes about
    dementia diagnosis, 14
  perspective of needs of primary care
    patients, 25–8
Geriatric Care Model, 5
Germany, 4, 5, 6, 29, 93
GPs. *see* general practitioners (GPs)
Groningen Activity Restriction Scale
    (GARS), 35–8

health inequalities, 1, 97, 98
hearing. *see* eyesight/hearing/
    communication needs
home treatment package for people
    with dementia
  development of, 65–72
  evaluation of, 72–3
  need for, 63–4
  preliminary work, 64–5
homeless population, 5–6
hospital admissions, prevention of, 62,
    63, 64, 73
hypertension, 28

India, 4
information needs
  of family carers, 54, 56, 99
  of people with dementia, 14, 16, 29,
    59
  of people living alone, 48
  of people with young-onset
    dementia, 79
  of primary care patients, 24

interventions for people with
    dementia, 64–5, 72, 73
  and case management, 63–4
  for family members, 82
  psychosocial interventions, 97–8
intimate relationships needs, 93
  of people with dementia, 15, 54, 88
  of people with depression, 6
  of people in long-term care, 87, 88
  of people in rural communities, 4
  of people with young-onset
    dementia, 79
  of primary care patients, 21
Iran, 4

Johns Hopkins Dementia Care Needs
    Assessment (JHDCNA), 11, 14

Korea, 4

Lebanon, 4
legal issues, 15, 16
living alone, 44–9
loneliness
  of people living alone, 44, 48
  of people with dementia, 15
  of spousal carers, 81
  risk factor for dementia and
    depression, 98
long-term care settings
  met and unmet needs, 88–9
  needs of general population, 87–8
  needs of people with dementia, 88
  overview of, 86–7
long-term conditions, 97, 98
looking after home needs
  of people with dementia, 48, 59
  of people in rural communities, 4
  of people living in residential homes,
    38
  of primary care patients, 21, 27, 28

major depressive illness, 6
Malaysia, 4
marital status as risk factor, 21, 87
memory needs
  impact on caregiver burden,
    56, 59
  of people with dementia, 29, 54
  of people with dementia living at
    home, 15, 59
  of people with dementia in long-
    term care, 88
  of people living alone, 48
Minimum Data Set for Home Care
    (MDS-HC), 5
mobility/falls needs, 21
  of people with dementia, 29, 59
  of people with depression, 6, 38
  of people in residential homes, 38

of people with young-onset
    dementia, 79–80
  of primary care patients, 20, 21, 24,
    25, 28
money/budgeting needs
  impact on caregiver burden, 56, 59
  of people with dementia, 54, 59
  of primary care patients, 25
musculoskeletal disorders, 20, 21, 24

needs assessment
  and community health, 5–6
  definition of, 1–2, 97
  difficulties due to mental illness and
    somatic disorders, 28–9
  discrepancies between needs
    reported by individuals, family
    carers and medical staff, 6, 20, 89
  engaging older people in, 98
  interrelatedness of needs, 14, 16
  and mental health, 6
  overview of older people's health
    needs, 1–2, 97
  research areas, 97–101
  and self-reported needs, 16
neglect. *see* abuse/neglect
Netherlands, 6, 34
  e-health programs, 82
  health care costs, 83
  studies of people with dementia, 3,
    56, 59, 78
  studies of primary care patients, 5,
    20
Norway, 77
Nottingham Health Needs Assessment
    (NHNA), 28
nutritional needs
  of people with dementia living alone,
    46
  of people with dementia living at
    home, 59
  of people with dementia in long-
    term care, 88
  of people in residential homes, 38

objective vs. subjective needs, 10

person-centred care, 10, 16–17, 138
pharmaceutical treatment
  non-pharmacological interventions,
    15, 16
  problem for people with dementia,
    15, 17
physical health needs
  of people with dementia living at
    home, 15–16, 17, 59
  of people with depression, 6
  of primary care patients, 20, 21, 24–6
Poland, 3–4
polymorbidity, 15, 16

polypharmacy, 15
Portugal, 3, 4, 6, 30
post-diagnostic support for dementia, 14–15
primary care patients, needs of, 20–31
    CANE adaptations for, 4, 5
    discrepancies between perspectives of individuals, relatives and GPs, 27–8, 29
    perspective of GPs, 25–8
    perspective of relatives, 25
    unmet needs, 24
psychological distress needs
    of family carers, 54, 56
    of people with dementia, 15, 16, 46, 59, 88
    of people with depression, 6, 38, 40
    of people in long-term care, 87
    of people in residential homes, 38
    of people with young-onset dementia, 78–9
    of primary care patients, 21, 24, 25, 27, 29
psychosocial needs. see also individual needs categories
    of people living alone, 49
    of people in long-term care, 87–8
psychotic symptoms needs
    of people with dementia living alone, 46
    of people with dementia in long-term care, 88
    of people with depression, 38, 40
    of people in residential homes, 38

quality of life
    definition of, 10
    of family carers, 59, 63
    and Geriatric Care Model, 5
    and health inequalities, 100
    and needs assessment, 1, 101

of people with dementia, 10, 16, 17, 62, 63, 64
of people with depression, 29, 34
of people in long-term care, 86, 87, 88
of people with mental illness, 6
of primary care patients, 30
Questionnaire for Health-Related Resource Use in an Elderly Population (FIMA), 92

research on needs assessment
    and clinical care, 99–100
    and family carers, 99
    and health of older people, 97–8
    and social health, 98
    and technology, 98–9
risk factors for unmet needs, 21, 30, 48
    for crises for people with dementia, 65
    for hospital admissions, 64
    for long-term care, 87

schizophrenia, 6
self-care needs, 48
self-harm (accidental), 16, 46, 48
self-harm (deliberate), 21, 54
sight. see eyesight/hearing/communication needs
sleep disorders, 100
social isolation
    of cardiac patients, 28, 29
    and intimate relationships needs, 93
    of people with dementia living at home, 15
    of people living alone, 44
    of people in rural communities, 4
    risk factor for dementia and depression, 98

social needs. see also company needs; daytime activities needs; intimate relationships needs
    of people with dementia living at home, 59
social roles, 15
SPICE assessment tool, 4, 30, 99
stroke aftercare, 4–5
subjective needs, 79, see also objective vs. subjective needs
suicidality, 29

technology, 98–9
Thailand, 4
Threshold Assessment Grid (TAG), 65

United Kingdom
    CANE studies in, 5, 6, 20, 57, 59
    demographic overview of dementia, 62
United Nations, 1
United States, 6, 44

wellbeing
    of carers, 63, 64, 97, 99
    of children of people with dementia, 81
    and healthy ageing, 97
    and needs assessment, 1, 10, 88
    of people with dementia, 10, 79, 97, 99
    of people living alone, 48
    and social health, 98

young-onset dementia
    needs of family members, 80–2
    needs of individuals, 78–80
    overview, 77–8
    use of CANE with care homes residents, 82–4